THE
COMPLETE
GUIDE TO
NUTRITIONAL
SUPPLEMENTS

THE
COMPLETE
GUIDE TO
NUTRITIONAL
SUPPLEMENTS

EVERYTHING YOU NEED TO MAKE INFORMED CHOICES FOR OPTIMUM HEALTH

Brenda D. Adderly, M.H.A.

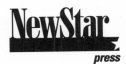

NewStar
press

ISBN: 0-7871-1769-2

NewStar Press
a division of NewStar Media Inc.
8955 Beverly Boulevard
Los Angeles, CA 90048

Cover design by Rick Penn-Kraus
Text design and layout by Carolyn Wendt
Printed by Victor Graphics

First NewStar Trade Paperback Printing: October 1998

10 9 8 7 6 5 4 3 2 1

Printed in the United States of America

PUBLISHER'S NOTE

The Complete Guide to Nutritional Supplements was compiled and written to provide an easy-to-read reference tool for consumers who want clear, concise information on the many nutritional supplements currently available. In doing so, we have assembled the best information and research currently available to help you in choosing the most appropriate supplement(s) to improve your health. This book, however, is designed to help you navigate the supplement aisles, not to be used as a recommendation of treatment or endorsement of any product.

The information contained in this book is not meant to take the place of any information provided by the product's maker, your physician, or other health care advisor, nor to substitute for any prescription that may be prescribed by your physician. If you suspect you have a medical problem or you have any questions regarding the safety or efficacy of any supplement or are being treated for any particular health condition, be sure to consult with your doctor or health practitioner before consuming any nutritional supplement.

The author and publisher disclaim any liability for any adverse effects resulting from the use of any information contained herein.

TABLE OF CONTENTS

FOREWORD

There has been an enormous change in medical care over the past few years. People nowadays want to take charge of their own health and stop relying completely on doctors to tell them what to do. Doctors used to have time to sit and talk about new strategies for keeping you in the best shape and treating illnesses with the fewest possible side effects. Unfortunately, doctors have less time now. Fortunately, you have this book, which will be a great source of information as you get more involved in keeping yourself healthy. Each page will make you feel more comfortable and confident about creating your own path toward optimal health.

Millions of people are now embracing alternatives in health care. A recent survey showed that well over 50 percent of the American public are using alternative medicine and wanted to know more about what they could do to empower themselves.

Every day of my career as a pediatrician, I've watched families use alternative medicine. I have received no formal training in alternative medicine but have learned much from my patients. I once prescribed antibiotics for a child with an ear infection and when the family returned for a checkup, I complimented them on their diligence in administering the gooey, unappealling prescription. "We didn't," they replied. When I asked them about their treatment, they told me about echinacea, homeopathy, garlic, and the like. I listened only a little. By the twentieth time this happened, I either had to listen closely and take notes or admit to being narrow-minded and not terribly scientific!

Recent medical research and numerous publications have validated the need to look for alternatives to antibiotics and other medications. You'll read about the remedies discussed in this book almost every day in your local newspaper for years to come.

Actually, you'll have information about the "newest" vitamin or supplement before the newspaper even reports it. As I read the last drafts of *The Complete Guide to Nutritional Supplements* to prepare for writing this, I learned something new each time through. Rest assured, you will too.

—*Jay N. Gordon, M.D., F.A.A.P.*

INTRODUCTION

Last night's news promises that you can "stop the clock" by using the newest, hottest nutritional supplement. Your best friend swears that a supplement relieved her PMS. Even your dad's in the game, telling you how some herb helped him improve his memory—and his golf game! All this sounds good, but what should you *really* believe?

Maybe you don't think you have an obvious need for supplementation right now. You're not sick. In fact, you look good, your energy is high, and you feel great.

Then you come down with the sniffles. You look in the medicine cabinet and there's nothing in there, so you bundle up and head to the store. You decide to go the natural route this time, because you don't want the side effects you had the last time you took a drug. But at the store you're faced with a seemingly endless aisle of nutritional supplements—all staring you down and intimidating you—with labels that give you half the information you need.

HOW TO USE THIS BOOK

The Complete Guide to Nutritional Supplements was created for you, the reader who is interested in using nutritional supplements but is confused by all the products available and the hype surrounding them. This might be your initial foray into using nutritional supplements, or you might already be quite knowledgeable and want a handy reference book to back up what you already know.

This book is the result of almost a year's worth of research, writing, compiling, and fact-checking. Health-care practitioners were consulted, publications and studies were reviewed and, in the process, the most definitive answers were sought out on the supplements referenced in this guide.

In doing my research for this book, I realized that quite a few of the supplements commonly used today have substantial research behind them. For many, costly studies have been conducted in Europe as well as in the United States. These studies have shown many of the supplements discussed here to be very effective for certain health conditions or for generally improving health.

In each entry, I have focused on the condition(s) for which the supplement is most commonly used. To alleviate any confusion over the supplements' proper usage, I have also listed the many other health concerns for which an individual supplement may be beneficial.

Certainly it's no wonder we're all confused. With hundreds of products, thousands of studies, and literally tons of allegations, how do you sift through the hype and get to the truth? The truth is relatively simple—and pretty positive: Most of the supplements on the market today *do* offer benefits. However, finding the one(s) right for you is the challenge.

But buyer, beware. It is important to understand the research behind the claims and to be able to distinguish what is clinically substantiated and what is not. For example, a nutritional supplement is tested and is found to be effective in treating heart conditions. Six months later you also hear that it's good for impotence, clear skin, and strengthening bones. How can you tell if the supplement really is effective for all that—or just for heart conditions?

This dilemma fuels my intent to educate consumers about the bewildering array of medical therapies and treatments available to us. Whether we are sick or want to maintain good health, we need accurate and reliable information that enables us to make the most appropriate decisions. Although it is always wise to consult a physician or licensed health-care practitioner in matters of our health and well being, we can't rely on these professionals completely. Taking an active role not only benefits us but also makes the job of the health professional more effective.

HOW THE SUPPLEMENTS ARE RATED

One thing that everyone can agree on today is that nutritional supplementation has value. What the value of each supplement is, and how it can best be used, are topics of endless discussion and speculation. Vitamins, minerals, and other supplements are not regulated by any U.S. agency, and therefore, no claims can be made by the makers. While this may protect the consumer from a host of unsubstantiated claims, it also adds to the widespread confusion. This confusion is why I chose to compile this book. Here, you will find a great deal of background information on each supplement: what works, what doesn't, and what *may* work for you. *The Complete Guide to Nutritional Supplements* then distills this information and research into three rating categories: Highly Recommended, Recommended, or Not Recommended.

- *Highly Recommended* indicates that at least five (5) conclusive studies have found the supplement to be an effective addition to a healthy diet and/or for specific health concerns.
- *Recommended* indicates that there are fewer than five conclusive studies, as well as some inconclusive studies, but that overwhelming clinical evidence supports the supplement.
- *Not Recommended* indicates that no conclusive studies were to be found, and clinical evidence is mixed. It may also indicate that no studies exist, just anecdotal evidence. There may be cases where this supplement offers benefits, however, with no strong research to support any claims, we do not recommend it.

What does the new RDI mean?

Since 1941, the Food and Nutrition Board of the National Research Council has been establishing the RDA, or Recommended Dietary Allowances, for vitamins and minerals. Originally, the RDA was designed to promote basic dietary completeness, and the amounts indicated as RDAs were considered the *minimum amount* necessary to prevent illness.

For many years now, RDAs have been criticized by the medical community as being a host of meaningless numbers. As more and more people have become proactive in dealing with their health, the Food and Nutrition Board has recognized that RDAs have been becoming less pertinent in people's lives. Acknowledging that today's Americans are more diverse and their needs do not easily fit into any one category, the Board began considering a new term: RDI, or Reference Dietary Intake.

The "Intake" amount will consider not only the amounts of vitamins and minerals needed to prevent disease but will also factor in the amounts necessary for good health. In 1998, this new system is in the process of being rolled out, and soon we will see RDIs completely replace RDAs.

While the RDI is an excellent starting place—and we have listed RDIs for the vitamins and minerals for which they have been established—please understand that your own specific needs may be significantly different from a figure established for the general population. Consider the RDI your starting point.

Under the Recommended Usage section of each entry, you will see the RDI amount. Directly following this amount are the suggested dosages that vary from the RDI for each particular health condition. While these numbers have been carefully researched and reported, supplements do not take the place of a healthy diet, hence the name *supplement*. In order to ensure the appropriate level of supplementation for your particular need, consult with a health-care practitioner.

Lifestyle factors, such as smoking and excessive alcohol consumption, should also be taken into account with the RDI. Because these deplete the body of necessary nutrients, check with your health-care provider to establish your particular supplement intake needs.

All in all, I know you'll find this book to be easy to read, clear to understand, and a handy reference to keep on hand when you visit your health food store or pharmacy. To keep up with the latest in natural treatments and therapies, stay in touch with me by regularly visiting my website at www.BrendaAdderly.com, or read my newsletter, *Health Watch*, for updates.

I'd love to hear from you and see how this book has helped you in your life.

To your health!

ACIDOPHILUS

Overall Rating . . . . *Highly Recommended*

To combat yeast infections . . . . *Highly Recommended*

To prevent urinary tract infections . . . *Highly Recommended*

To alleviate digestive disorders . . . . . . *Recommended*

To aid digestion in the
lactose intolerant . . . . *Recommended*

For healthy skin . . . . *Not Recommended*

To lower cholesterol . . . . *Recommended*

To reduce the odds of breast cancer . . . *Recommended*

There are places south of the equator—particularly the rain forests—where flora grows lush and wild and fast. Blaze a trail today, and by morning it'll be overgrown. Curiously, a similar ecosystem thrives in our intestines. This inner jungle consists of intestinal flora, a collection of bacteria and microorganisms that keep the intestines clean and prevent disease-carrying pathogens from making themselves at home. A major portion of this amiable bacteria is acidophilus, more formally termed *Lactobacillus acidophilus*.

Acidophilus is a probiotic—kind of the opposite of an antibiotic, because probiotics keep (helpful) bacteria alive. In fact, acidophilus is often prescribed (along with its counterpart, bifidobacteria) in conjunction with long courses of antibiotics to alleviate side effects such as diarrhea and growth of the fungus

Monilia abricans, which grows in the intestines and vagina and also causes a white film in the mouth known as thrush. These side effects occur because antibiotics destroy the good bacteria along with the bad, and acidophilus helps by building our good guys back up again. Acidophilus also kills other types of yeast and fungi on contact and is particularly helpful in combating *Candida albicans,* the culprit in most vaginal yeast infections, says William Crook, M.D., author of *The Yeast Connection.* Women with frequent yeast infections are thought to gain some relief by eating a daily cup of yogurt, which is rich in acidophilus culture.

There are many benefits from taking acidophilus. It can be found in yogurt, milk, kefir, and various soy products. Acidophilus is thought to

- treat and prevent vaginal yeast infections and ward off recurring urinary tract infections, according to Michael Murray, N.D., and Joseph Pizzorno, N.D., authors of *Encyclopedia of Natural Medicine*
- get rid of chronic bad breath that won't respond to mouthwash
- reduce constipation and gas
- promote healthy skin
- potentially help people with lactose deficiency digest milk products

Acidophilus is also thought to hamper cancerous cells from forming in the intestines and colon and to lower cholesterol in those who consume it regularly, according to several studies conducted by the U.S. Dairy Farmers Association. Another important cancer-related study published by *The American Journal of Clinical Nutrition* indicates that hyperestrogenism and possibly breast cancer itself may be decreased by ingesting acidophilus, because the bacteria helps to metabolize estrogen properly.

In addition to its prevalence in yogurt and milk, acidophilus is available as a supplement in both liquid and capsule form. And if you're up for a challenge, a fun way to "home grow" acidophilus is to make your own yogurt.

 ## RECOMMENDED USAGE

There is no RDI for acidophilus.

Children
Administer with the advice of a doctor or health practitioner.

Adults
Two 500-milligram capsules three times daily with meals.

 ## CAUTION!

Intestinal flora are very important to maintaining a healthy immune system. When these helpful bacteria are destroyed, our bodies are left vulnerable to the clamor of harmful bacteria that want to grow in their place. Because antibiotics will destroy intestinal flora, anyone taking a high dose of antibiotics might want to use acidophilus supplements until the medication has run its course. Also of note: Without lactic acid or lactose, these friendly bugs can only survive for about a week. If acidophilus products don't appeal to you, other substances that help intestinal flora grow include vitamin C, complex carbohydrates, and pectin.

Acidophilus culture is not known to be toxic, but anyone with intestinal problems should check with a doctor before adding it to their diet or program of supplements. This is also true for people who suffer from vaginal yeast infections and urinary tract infections. Even though acidophilus can benefit these conditions, it's a good idea to seek outside medical treatment in addition to using the supplement. Finally, women who want to apply acidophilus vaginally should do so only under professional supervision.

ALFALFA
(*Medicago sativa*)

Overall Rating . . . . *Highly Recommended*

To promote calcium absorption . . . . . *Highly Recommended*

To reduce cholesterol . . . . *Recommended*

For breastfeeding women . . . . *Recommended*

What's small, green, crunchy, and one of the most potent multivitamin supplements you can take? You guessed it: the alfalfa sprout! The darling of the health food set, who don't mind eating something with a funny texture, alfalfa contains significant amounts of vitamins A, B, C, E, and K; protein; a variety of essential minerals; enzymes; and calcium. In fact, 1 ounce of alfalfa powder contains 75 percent of the recommended daily intake (RDI) of calcium—important news for women over age forty-five who are at risk for osteoporosis. Plus the vitamin K in alfalfa promotes calcium absorption, so there's no doubt the calcium you're eating will actually make it to your bones.

Remarkably, alfalfa, which sometimes masquerades under the more sophisticated name lucerne, was reported in the scientific journal *Atherosclerosis* to successfully reduce cholesterol. Because of its other nutritious properties, it can also

- prevent plaque buildup in arteries
- guard against stroke
- promote blood clotting
- prevent hemorrhaging

No wonder alfalfa is a primary feed for cattle. According to a recent study reported in *Mothering*, not only does it provide all those essential nutrients, it also increases milk supply. Nursing mothers seeking to do the same can blend alfalfa tea with herbs such as fennel, fenugreek, and dandelion, and end up with good results.

Folk remedies call for applying alfalfa juice to open wounds to prevent infection or brushing teeth with a peeled alfalfa root.

Alfalfa sprouts are commonly found in the supermarket produce section. They are also easy to grow at home. Simply soak alfalfa seeds for several hours, and then place them in a glass jar with cheesecloth or mesh sealing the top. Put the jar in a dark place. Wash and drain the seeds each day, and after three or four days you'll have plenty of nutritious sprouts for your sandwiches and salads.

 ## RECOMMENDED USAGE

There is no RDI for alfalfa.

Children
Children can safely eat alfalfa sprouts. Supplements should be administered only under the advice of a doctor or health practitioner.

Adults
Alfalfa tea, tablets, and powder are available at most health food stores. To help lower cholesterol, try taking 40 grams of alfalfa seeds three times a day for eight weeks.

For general purposes, eat the sprouts as part of your regular diet, or take tablets as instructed on the container label.

The tea is especially delicious with honey and lemon or orange rind.

CAUTION!

If you have lupus or another autoimmune disease, do not use alfalfa in any form. A compound in the plant could trigger a dangerous response.

ALOE VERA

Overall Rating . . . . *Highly Recommended*

For healing burns,
including sunburn . . . . *Highly Recommended*

For healing cuts,
and other skin repair . . . . *Highly Recommended*

For overall skin conditioning . . . . *Recommended*

To relieve constipation . . . . *Recommended*

Trace the medicinal uses of the aloe vera plant through time, and you'll end up zigzagging from tropical Africa, to Egypt, Greece, and Rome. In the south of Africa—where aloe comes from—whenever someone got hit with a poison arrow, the thick gel inside the plant's leaves would be employed to heal the wound. Farther north, Egyptians are thought to have used aloe during the embalming process. Perhaps that's what gave their famously vain queen, Cleopatra, the idea to use the gel on her face to preserve her girlish looks and protect her skin from the brutal desert sun. The Romans and Greeks, renowned for their wars, also sought the help of aloe for battle wounds, while in the Middle Ages, aloe gel and juice were ingested as purgatives.

These days, the uses of aloe vera gel continue to be pretty impressive. In the last three years alone, aloe has been incorporated into the list of pharmaceutical "must haves" in American hospitals, largely due to an extensive research study in Thailand that proved its properties relieve the pain, blistering, and peeling of burns—including sunburn and burns from radiation associated with cancer treatments. In addition, the study showed that the use of aloe sped up the healing process by almost 25 percent.

We can benefit from this yuccalike plant for

- speedy aid to cuts and insect bites
- moisturizing dry skin and hair, or softening calluses and corns
- easing constipation (without upsetting the stomach)
- potentially boosting the immune system

Surely by now you've learned that aloe vera is good for the skin. That's because it contains properties that actually kill pain, reduce inflammation, and prevent histamine reactions resulting in irritated, itchy skin. In fact, a landmark 1996 study published in *Ethnopharmacology* underscores the important anti-inflammatory properties of aloe. But if you've used it only for troublesome skin conditions, you're missing out on some of its other, more wide-ranging benefits.

Current research published in the trade journal *Pharmacology* indicates that, taken internally in the form of gel or juice, the aloe extract Carrisyn may actually fight viral infections. Preliminary test tube studies performed in Germany show that Carrisyn may even prevent the reproduction of viruses such as HIV and herpes. This unique element also seems to incite our immune systems to build more T cells and other protective substances.

Because aloe has for so long been used for its medicinal effects, lots of proactive, though unproven benefits have surfaced. Drinking it might just arouse your appetite and your sex drive. It's also been used to reactivate a woman's menstrual cycles. Men and women alike may relieve headaches by applying the cool plant to the head. When inhaled within steam, aloe may clean clogged bronchial tubes.

This beneficial substance can be purchased in several forms. Most health food stores and pharmacies sell aloe vera gel and juice, while nurseries everywhere sell aloe plants for the home. When buying the gel, be sure it's at least 97 percent pure and aloe is listed at the top of the ingredients. Otherwise you might get stuck with something that doesn't really help.

Having an aloe plant on hand is especially helpful for those everyday burns and irritations. Just cut off a part of the leaf and apply the gel directly to the spot that hurts. If there's a bit of the leaf leftover, don't throw it away. Simply wrap it in foil and put it in the fridge. Fresh aloe does best when kept cool and dry—but don't go overboard and freeze it. Once frozen it doesn't revive.

 ## RECOMMENDED USAGE

There is no RDI for aloe vera.

Adults and Children
For topical use
Use on skin as needed to moisturize or relieve pain.

Adults
For internal use
One 100-milligram capsule up to three times daily.
Consult your doctor or health practitioner before taking aloe internally.

 ## CAUTION!

Aloe vera is nontoxic and thought to be safe when taken in moderation. Because the aloe plant acts as such a strong purgative, however, it's not recommended for pregnant women. If after drinking aloe vera gel or juice you encounter nausea, vomiting, abdominal cramps, or diarrhea, discontinue immediately and seek the assistance of a health-care practitioner.

For some people, applying aloe vera gel externally may cause an allergic reaction such as redness, itching, and hives. If this happens to you, it's wise to discontinue using aloe products.

ARGININE

Overall Rating. . . . . *Recommended*

To boost the immune system . . . . *Recommended*

Unlike the other nonessential aminos, arginine can become essential for those who've suffered some kind of physical trauma. That's because arginine strengthens the immune system by making infection-fighting lymphocytes. In fortifying the immune system, arginine also may

- slow tumor growth and recurrence
- speed up the healing of wounds and burns
- detoxify the liver
- prevent loss of muscle after injury or surgery.

Because arginine incites the pituitary gland to release Growth Hormone (GH), some people claim it burns fat and builds muscle, though this is unsubstantiated. GH is believed to be related, however, to arginine's ability to help heal wounds quickly. This amino acid also helps regulate normal sperm production. In a recent Norwegian study, supplementation resulted in increased sperm counts.

 RECOMMENDED USAGE

There is no RDI for arginine.

Children
Administer only under the advice of a doctor or health practitioner.

Adults

Capsules

One 100-milligram capsule up to three times daily.

 CAUTION!

Because it stimulates the release of Growth Hormone, arginine supplements should not be given to children as it could affect their proper growth rate. Arginine in high doses may also cause nausea, diarrhea, and a thickening of the skin, as well as agitation of your mental state or metabolism. If these symptoms occur, stop taking supplements and see a health practitioner.

A debate also exists as to whether or not arginine makes people with herpes more susceptible to outbreaks. To date, this has not been substantiated but is something to take into consideration when supplementing your diet.

Arginine is not recommended for anyone diagnosed with kidney or liver failure.

ARNICA
(*Arnica montana*)

Overall Recommendation. . . . . *Recommended*

For reducing skin pain and irritations . . . . . . *Recommended*

To relieve muscle soreness and pain . . . . *Recommended*

Throughout time, arnica has been successfully used in many ways. Native Americans used it as a pain reliever and a stimulant and for skin irritations.

Topically, arnica can relieve the symptoms of osteoarthritis and muscle soreness. In fact, numerous clinical studies and personal anecdotes report that homeopathic arnica gel or cream, rubbed directly on the sore area, relieves the discomfort. Arnica is also considered helpful in the healing of bruises and muscle strains.

However, because of its high toxicity when ingested, naturopaths, homeopaths, and herbalists recommend that arnica be used only on the skin, unless administered and supervised by a doctor or health practitioner.

 ## RECOMMENDED USAGE

There is no RDI for arnica.

Use arnica cream or salve topically as needed for aches and pains.

Not advised for pregnant or lactating women.

CAUTION!

Taken internally, arnica is easy to overdose on and can be fatal. Do not take unless administered by your doctor or health practitioner.
Do not apply arnica to broken or bleeding skin.

ASTRAGALUS

Overall Rating . . . . *Recommended*

To improve immune function . . . . *Highly Recommended*
For alleviating symptoms of the
common cold. . . . . *Highly Recommended*

A very common supplement in traditional Chinese medicine, astragalus root has been used for hundreds of years to treat viral infections and the common cold. Its stellar results were studied and reported over a decade ago in *Pharmacology and Applications of Chinese Materia Medica*. That information has since mainstreamed into the American culture, and astragalus has become one of the top supplements in today's herbal combination formulas.

Extensive research with animals and humans has shown that astragalus is a strong booster of the immune system. These studies indicate that astragalus works by stimulating the body's sluggish parts, thus allowing the body to rejuvenate itself. This theory has been so well tested in China that doctors there commonly prescribe astragalus to their patients following cancer chemotherapy treatments.

 RECOMMENDED USAGE

There is no RDI for astragalus.

Children

Not advised for children. Administer only under the advice of a doctor or health practitioner.

Adults

Capsules

One 100-milligram capsule up to three times daily.

Tincture

Three drops in an 8-ounce glass of water three times daily.

BILBERRY
(*Vaccinum myrtillus*)

Overall Rating . . . . *Recommended*

To reduce inflammation . . . . *Recommended*

For treating digestive disorders . . . . *Recommended*

Never heard of bilberries? That's okay—chances are you've eaten cup after cup of them in muffins, pies, over ice cream, or picked fresh from what you called a blueberry or huckleberry bush. Although some botanists believe that bilberries, cowberries, and blueberries are the same berry, others think that they are just very close cousins. It doesn't matter who's right, because all these berries deliver essentially the same health benefits. (They taste great, too!)

Bilberries are one of those wonderful foods that have few calories but provide a load of nutrition. One cup of bilberries contains almost one third of the RDI for vitamin C, and good doses of potassium and pectin, a dietary fiber. They're also full of flavonoids and anti-inflammatory properties.

Vitamin C, you may recall, is an antioxidant that helps your body fight infection and keeps your blood vessels nice and clean. That means less possibility of clogged arteries that can lead to heart attack or stroke. Potassium keeps bodily fluids in balance and works to normalize heart function and blood pressure. Pectin may help lower cholesterol levels. So next time your mouth waters for a fresh blueberry muffin from your favorite bakery, you have every reason to go for it!

According to *Biochemical Pharmacology*, the berries' anti-inflammatory qualities can help people with rheumatoid arthritis. All that's necessary is a liberal handful applied straight to the mouth on a regular basis.

If you commonly experience tired eyes or realize your night vision isn't as good as it used to be, try eating a ½ cup of fresh or frozen blueberries each day. Besides tasting good, they just might help prevent vision disorders such as cataracts and macular degeneration.

Bilberries are a proven remedy for diarrhea. But beware: eating too many will have the opposite effect. And lest you think the berry is the only useful part of the plant, bilberry leaf tea can be used as a mouthwash to soothe sore gums or combined with witch hazel to wash over sunburn, eczema, or burns. Drinking bilberry leaf tea is thought to aid in healing ulcers and may, by lowering blood sugar, help offset the symptoms of late-onset noninsulin-dependent diabetes.

 RECOMMENDED USAGE

There is no RDI for bilberries.

Children
Supplementation not advised for children. Administer only under the advice of a doctor or health practitioner.

Adults
Capsules
One to two 40-milligram capsules up to three times daily.
Tincture
Three drops in an 8-ounce glass of water three times daily.

While you may have to visit your health food store to find bilberry powder or tea, the benefits of the berries themselves are as close as your supermarket. Blueberry pies, muffins, ice cream—and, of course, the fresh berries—can all provide medicinal results.

For constipation, eat a large bowl of berries.

Drinking 10 milliliters of unsweetened juice best treats diarrhea. Start with one glass and if that doesn't do the trick, drink another. For chronic diarrhea, make a decoction of tea and take it daily.

 CAUTION!

People suffering from late-onset (noninsulin dependent) diabetes should consult with a health professional before using bilberries to ease their symptoms. Similarly, people with kidney problems should use bilberries with caution because of their high potassium content.

BIOFLAVONOIDS
(a.k.a. Flavonoids)

Overall Rating . . . . *Highly Recommended*

To increase circulation . . . . *Highly Recommended*
To reduce the likelihood of cancers. . . *Recommended*
To reduce allergies . . . . *Recommended*
For increasing bone density . . . . *Highly Recommended*

If you "bruise like a peach" or suffer from bleeding gums, bioflavonoids—also known as flavonoids or vitamin P—might go a long way to strengthening your capillaries and connective tissues. The primary functions of flavonoids are to prevent circulatory problems, including heart disease, bruising, and varicose veins, and to assist in the absorption of vitamin C. While you're at it, enlisting the help of these antioxidant powerhouses may also help you to

* ward off viral infections
* prevent lung and prostate cancer
* reduce swelling and allergic reactions, including asthma
* improve eyesight.

The very popular journal *Cancer Letter* reported that the incidence of all cancers—and lung and prostate cancers in particular—were reduced when dietary supplements of flavonoids were taken. In addition, those with concerns of osteoporosis or bone healing should supplement with flavonoids, according to a long-term Swedish study.

Flavonoids are such a large and unique group of nutrients that not all of them have been identified. And although many flavonoids have been used for their medicinal properties for centuries in Chinese herbs such as Sho-saiko-to, Western medicine has not yet considered them important enough to officially label them vitamins—which is why vitamin P may sound unfamiliar.

Even so, we can thank flavonoids for the zest they bring to mealtime because they color and flavor fruits and vegetables. And it is in those foods that they are most abundant. They can be found in other foods containing vitamin C, because they protect it from oxidation.

The flavonoids that keep us from bruising when we bump into things mainly include rutin, hesperidin, and proanthocyanidin, which can be found in citrus fruits (especially in the pulp and rind), red wine, berries, buckwheat, and pine bark.

And for the days when we are particularly clumsy, the flavonoid quercetin, found in onions and garlic, reduces inflammation and swelling, according to several recent double-blind studies. But quercetin not only helps reduce the swelling associated with klutziness, it's great for agitated bronchial tubes as well. That's because it's thought to act as an antidote against allergic reactions, which makes it an effective treatment both for hay fever and asthma, according to recent studies conducted in Sweden on bioflavonoids. And although quercetin alone may help your body fight viruses and cancer, a unique property of garlic known as allicin boosts this potential. All that, plus it's an antioxidant!

On one of your more graceful days, you might try cooking with the yellow spice turmeric, popular in Indian foods. By doing so, you'll reap the benefits of the flavonoid curcumin, which helps conditions ranging from arthritis to asthma. It, like all the other flavonoids, has antioxidant properties that protect us from cancer and heart disease.

If Indian food doesn't excite you, there are plenty of other antioxidant-rich foods filled with flavonoids, including alfalfa sprouts, broccoli, brussel sprouts, garlic, kale, spinach, apricots, blueberries, carrots, cantaloupes, grains, legumes, mangos, nuts, papaya, red and green peppers, seeds, squash, sweet potatoes, tomatoes, and watermelons, even coffee, green tea, and the herb gingko biloba.

Luckily, getting your flavonoids is as simple as maintaining a diet rich in fruits and vegetables. If you're like some of us, however, and prefer to fill up on chips instead of fruits during snack time, you might want to boost your flavonoid intake with supplements. Be sure to take them. That way you get the benefits of flavonoids while increasing your body's ability to absorb that much-needed vitamin C.

 ## RECOMMENDED USAGE

There is no RDI for flavonoids.

Children
Administer only under the advice of a doctor or health practitioner.

Adults
Dosages range by flavonoid compound:
Quercetin: 200–400 milligrams three times daily
Citrus bioflavonoids: 1,000–3,000 milligrams daily

 ## CAUTION!

One of the primary functions of flavonoids is to reduce bleeding gums. But if you have persistent bleeding, be sure to consult your physician before using flavonoids as a remedy. That way you can prevent the possibility of masking a more serious condition.

Fruits and vegetables are known for their healthful properties. But if certain ones agitate your system, you might have a food allergy and should contact your physician. The good news is that if you do have a food allergy, flavonoids are in such a wide variety of foods, you'll most likely find a source that works for you.

As far as we know, flavonoids have no adverse effects on the body. Even so, take supplements in conjunction with a good dose of common sense.

BIOTIN

Overall Rating . . . . *Recommended*

To promote fat metabolism . . . . *Recommended*

To alleviate skin conditions . . . . *Recommended*

For healthy hair . . . . *Recommended*

For preventing hair loss . . . . *Not Recommended*

To help treat diabetes. . . . . *Highly Recommended*

Think of one of the best meals you've had at your favorite Italian bistro. It begins with a glass of merlot (good for cleaning up our fast-food arteries), home-baked foccacia bread drizzled in olive oil (proven to be the healthiest of all oils), and a Caesar salad heaped with freshly grated Parmesan cheese (calcium, lots of calcium!). These appetizers are just the beginning of an enormous feast. The meal goes on all night, and afterward, on the wobble home, you may feel that your soul has been fed—but what have you really done to your body?

It's truly unfair that some of the most delicious foods are less than good for us, but at least biotin helps us make the most of whatever we eat. A member of the B-complex family, biotin is a coenzyme that's made by bacteria in the intestines. When the carbohydrates, fats, and protein from our foods come down the pike, biotin is waiting to massage them into shape so that our bodies can put them to use. Without enough biotin, fat metabolism can be impaired and cholesterol levels go up.

Biotin is most popularly known for its vital role in maintaining healthy hair and skin. According to a multitude of dermatologic studies conducted in the United States and abroad, it alleviates skin conditions such as eczema and dermatitis. The newborn version of these skin conditions is cradle cap, characterized by a red and itchy scalp. Because babies don't have the intestinal bacteria needed to make biotin, supplements are sometimes employed to bring them relief and, according to Japanese researchers, have produced good results. Furthermore, biotin can help tame stubborn cowlicks—otherwise known as "uncombable hair syndrome"—in children. Of course, anyone thinking about biotin supplements for their child should be sure to play it safe and first check with a pediatrician.

For those who struggle not with combing hair but with having no hair to comb, biotin is often touted as being able to reverse balding or to prevent what hair you have from turning gray. Unfortunately, such claims have not been proven. Biotin supplements help hair grow back only if it's falling out because of the body's lack of biotin.

Biotin has also been found to enhance insulin sensitivity and encourage the liver to utilize glucose more efficiently. This is an important consideration in treating diabetes, reported a study in the medical journal *Life Sciences*.

Most of the biotin in our bodies is made internally, but we can also get it from a number of foods. The two richest biotin food sources are beef liver and brewer's yeast. But if these choices don't score high with your taste buds, other sources include bananas, cheese, chicken, cooked eggs, lamb, milk, oatmeal, peanut butter, pork, rice, soybeans, and whole-wheat flour.

RDI

Children
20–100 micrograms
Nonbreast-fed infants: 100–300 micrograms

Adults
25–50 years: 300 micrograms
50+ years: 300 micrograms

Rather than purchasing a separate supplement, biotin is easily found in B-complex and multivitamin supplements.

 CAUTION!

It's rare that someone will naturally suffer from a biotin deficiency, as most result from ingesting foods and substances that prevent biotin from doing its job. Biotin blockers include tobacco smoking, long courses of antibiotics, and excessive amounts of raw egg whites (say, nearly two dozen a day—easy to consume if you're drinking several very high protein smoothies a day, as many bodybuilders do). People who are on extremely low calorie diets—including anorexics—are also at risk for having low biotin. Of course in these instances, biotin supplementation isn't the only solution—caloric uptake is also necessary for optimum health.

Telltale signs of biotin deficiency may include eczema, increased cholesterol levels, hair loss, depression, and fatigue. If you feel your biotin may be low, supplements are a safe choice. As helpful as this little coenzyme is for your body, it's also harmless and nontoxic. So if you take more biotin than you really need, your body will simply dispose of it.

BLUE-GREEN ALGAE

Overall Rating . . . . *Not Recommended*

To increase energy and stamina . . . . *Not Recommended*
For greater mental capacity . . . . *Not Recommended*

Imagine a supplement made from what looks like pond scum. Interested? Probably not. Now imagine this: What if that pond scum were full of protein, vitamin B_{12}, beta-carotene, chlorophyll, amino acids, linolenic acid, nucleic acid, and minerals? Interested now? Probably more so. Claims for blue-green algae state that if you just sprinkle some of this freeze-dried powder into your morning smoothie, you'll get all these nutrients. That's pretty much the idea behind blue-green algae.

Although it has not been proven and very little research has been conducted, people claim that by adding blue-green algae to their diet on a regular basis, it can boost energy, stimulate the immune system, improve mental clarity, increase sexual stamina, alleviate thyroid problems, improve iron levels in blood, successfully treat hypoglycemia, improve digestion, combat allergies, and suppress the appetite, among other things.

Generally speaking, blue-green algae has been called "brain food," with properties that, absorbed by the body, can enable the body to heal itself. Pretty impressive claims for a substance that is at the very bottom of the food chain! Unfortunately, studies reveal that many of the claims made are just that: claims. And while anecdotal evidence is favorable, there is no science to substantiate those claims.

RECOMMENDED USAGE

There is no RDI for blue-green algae.

Children
Not advised for children. Administer only under the advice of a doctor or health practitioner.

Adults
You can find this product in drug and health food stores or through distributors on the Internet. Use as directed. Adults may take up to four 250-milligram capsules daily between meals.

 ## CAUTION!

Some people may experience side effects when taking blue-green algae, such as nausea, vomiting, weakness, and numbness of extremities. Discontinue use immediately if any of these occur, and call a health-care practitioner.

Studies of the effect of blue-green algae on laboratory rats noted the rats suddenly being unable to breathe. Nevertheless, the Food and Drug Administration (FDA) has never found toxins in the substances fed to humans, nor have there been reports of humans having such severe reactions. However, exercise caution when using this product since little is known about it.

BORAGE

Overall Rating . . . . *Highly Recommended*

For reducing depression and anxiety . . . *Recommended*

For relieving arthritis . . . . *Highly Recommended*

To alleviate skin conditions . . . . *Highly Recommended*

To help combat PMS . . . . *Highly Recommended*

To ease hangovers . . . . *Not Recommended*

Also: Excellent source of omega-6 fatty acids

When things got dull in medieval times, folks would take in a tournament to watch the strongest men in the land fight to the death. And while preparing for a good joust, the nervous competitors would often drink a cup of borage tea to give them courage—which, in fact, it did. That's because the leaves of this lavender-flowered herb can excite our adrenal glands and get our adrenaline flowing. These days, however, borage seeds are causing all the stir, because when compressed they form borage oil, a major source of gamma linolenic acid (GLA), an essential fatty acid. This oil is useful for a number of reasons because it is thought to

- ✿ reduce the symptoms of arthritis
- ✿ help control menstruation, potentially relieving PMS
- ✿ soothe and clear up eczema
- ✿ possibly ease hangover distress

According to a recent German study involving borage oil's effect on arthritis, when used over time, it can lessen the swelling, stiffness, and constant ache of rheumatoid arthritis. And because it's natural, borage oil doesn't have the side effects of most prescription medications used to alleviate arthritis pain. Borage oil may also be used as an alternative to evening primrose oil for women seeking relief from the physical and emotional symptoms of premenstrual syndrome, says Christiane Northrup, M.D., author of the landmark book *Women's Bodies, Women's Wisdom*.

If you're breastfeeding, these coarse, dark-green leaves are thought to increase the milk flow. Or if you've been feeling blue, bloated, or itchy, they may also lift depression and anxiety, reduce water retention, rejuvenate dry skin, and help your body get back in balance after steroid therapy. In the past, the flowers of the borage plant were used in cough syrups, and in conjunction with the leaves, they can bring relief for both dry coughs and pleurisy.

Borage oil can most easily be found in the form of capsules, while leaf extracts are sold in tinctures.

 ## RECOMMENDED USAGE

There is no RDI for borage.

Children
Administer only under the advice of a doctor or health practitioner.

Adults
One 200-milligram capsule three times daily.
Three drops of the tincture in an 8-ounce glass of water three times daily.

☠ CAUTION!

Even though deficiency symptoms for borage haven't been defined for the general population, deficiency guidelines do exist for people who are low on essential fatty acids.

Overall, borage is nontoxic. The oil, however, should be taken in doses lower than 800 milligrams per day. Anything over that amount should be supervised by a health professional. The reason is that too much gamma linolenic acid, which is found in borage oil, may upset your balance of fatty acids.

Furthermore, as with all omega-6 fatty acids, borage oil is most appropriate for people who do not have high blood cholesterol.

ESSENTIAL FATTY ACIDS
(Omega-3 & Omega-6)

The story of the essential fatty acids is recognizable in all our favorite tales of martyrs. Blamed for all that was wrong in the world, they were despised, abused, and run out of town. Then one day, some wise and generous souls recognized their worth, spread the word, and suddenly they found themselves invited to a hero's return.

The moral of the story: Not all fat is bad. That's because the essential fatty acids (EFAs), gleaned mostly from plant foods, cold-water fish, and herbs, play a huge role in maintaining our health. But unlike so many other properties that help make us tick, they have to be gotten from diet because we're not able to make them within our bodies.

Essential fatty acids are broken down into two groups: the

omega-3s and the omega-6s. Both groups help create prostaglandins, substances akin to hormones, which govern all our major systems: cardiovascular, immune, nervous, and reproductive. EFAs also help construct the membranes of every cell in our body, basically by standing guard, deciding what substances go in and out of the cell, and ultimately protecting it from harmful invaders. These remarkable nutrients are also thought to fight cancer and slow the effects of multiple sclerosis, while also keeping our skin supple and glowing.

Omega-3 fatty acids are composed of linolenic acid and produce anti-inflammatory prostaglandins, which can help prevent cancerous cells from spreading; keep arteries from hardening by thinning the blood (just like aspirin only without the stomach upset); lower blood pressure; relieve angina-related chest pains; reduce symptoms of allergic conditions such as asthma, gout, and psoriasis by blocking prostaglandins that cause inflammation; and may help treat mental disorders such as schizophrenia and manic depression.

Omega-3's linolenic acid is derived from three substances: alpha-linolenic acid (LNA), eicosapentenoic acid (EPA), and docosahexanoic acid (DHA). Flaxseed oil provides the most abundant source of LNA, but it's hard to keep fresh, and smoking, drinking, and some medications may prevent it from being properly converted in the body (see Flaxseed Oil). It may be simpler to rely on eating nuts or cooking with canola or soybean oil for adequate amounts of LNA.

Eskimos are hale, hearty, and healthy because of the fish they eat, which is rich in EPA and DHA. But you don't have to move to Alaska to be as healthy as them. Just "fish" through those cookbooks for some cod, herring, mackerel, tuna, sardine, or salmon recipes. They'll do plenty to stimulate your health as well as your taste buds.

Although both are composed of linoleic acid, the omega-6 fatty acids differ from the omega-3s in that they produce different kinds of anti-inflammatory prostaglandins as well as some pro-inflammatory prostaglandins. Like omega-3s, omega-6 fatty acids are good for the heart because they help thin blood and reduce chest pains related to angina. They are also thought to prevent or stop the growth of cancerous tumors; stop the pain and inflammation of arthritis, eczema, and dermatitis; relieve symptoms of premenstrual syndrome; block pro-inflammatory prostaglandins in the uterus that cause painful menstrual periods; when taken with vitamin E, help diabetics normalize fat imbalances; increase fat metabolism, potentially leading to weight loss; help treat mental disorders, such as schizophrenia and hyperactivity, in children.

Linoleic acid, cis-linoleic acid, and gamma-linoleic acid (GLA) make up the omega-6s and are most abundant in plants and vegetable oils. Good sources for omega-6 fatty acids are in the oils of corn, canola, borage, black currant, and evening primrose. Of the three omega-6 substances, GLA—most prevalent in borage and black currant oil—is thought to be the most beneficial. Beware that corn, canola, and evening primrose oil contain high amounts of linoleic acid, which produces pro-inflammatory prostaglandins.

If this sounds a little too complicated, simply eat cold-water fish three times a week and take an occasional dose of borage oil.

All the essential fatty acids are available in supplemental form. If you decide to take omega-3 EPA and DHA supplements (most often found in fish oil capsules), be sure vitamin E is listed as one of the ingredients. It's the E that prevents the oil from going bad. Better yet, take a vitamin E supplement in conjunction with fish oil capsules to keep them from oxidizing in the body.

BORON

Overall Rating . . . . *Highly Recommended*

For increasing bone density . . . . *Highly Recommended*

For preventing osteoporosis . . . . *Recommended*

To reduce symptoms of osteoarthritis . . *Recommended*

When most people think about what it takes to keep their bones healthy and strong, calcium pops to mind. And for good reason. But that's not the only substance that keeps us upright and firm: Recent American studies published in *Environmental Health Perspective* show that the trace mineral boron works with calcium, vitamin D, and magnesium to help bones grow, stay strong, and even heal more quickly after fractures. All this contributes to good defense against osteoporosis.

Boron is an important player in the business of healthy bones because, according to a 1990 study that monitored the interrelationship between boron, magnesium, and bone strength, it promotes both the absorption and retention of calcium and magnesium within the bones and it reduces the loss of calcium through the urine. Hence, less bone loss and demineralization. In fact, boron's impact so significantly reduces the opportunity for osteoporosis in older women that it may soon be considered a natural and less harmful alternative to estrogen replacement therapy (ERT).

While boron bustles around inside our bones, it also appears to affect joints. Some research indicates that boron improves your body's anti-inflammatory abilities and may therefore help reduce the pain and swelling of arthritis, according to ongoing studies in Germany that have used boron supplementation to study its effects on joint health.

Eating plenty of fruits and vegetables probably supplies most of us with enough boron to pump up our bones. That means consuming apples, beans, dates, grapes, peaches, and pears. But don't go looking for boron in beef, chicken, or fish—you won't find much there.

 RDI

Children
Administer only under the advice of a doctor or health practitioner.

Adults
Capsules or tablets: 3 milligrams daily
For arthritis or osteoporosis: 9 milligrams daily

Although boron has been around forever, it's really just arrived on the nutrition scene in the past decade. As of yet, neither RDIs nor symptoms of boron deficiency have been determined. However, most nutritional experts suggest you get 3 milligrams of boron per day. Furthermore, people who suffer from osteoporosis and arthritis tend to be low on boron and could benefit from a supplemental dose of up to 9 milligrams daily.

If you don't feel you get enough boron from your food (a healthy diet of fruits and vegetables will most likely provide close to 2.5 milligrams daily), supplements are available as sodium borate. A multivitamin enhanced with boron, however, will probably meet your needs.

CAUTION!

Boron research is just beginning, so toxicity levels are as yet undetermined. As there have been no harmful side effects for people taking doses from 3 to 9 milligrams, you should not exceed that amount.

BREWER'S YEAST

Overall Rating . . . . *Highly Recommended*

For healing wounds . . . . *Recommended*

To help ward off fleas (pets only) . . . . *Recommended*

Any animal lover knows how hard it is when their furry friend becomes infested with fleas. There are chemically treated collars that help—but there's also an organic, nontoxic remedy to alleviate the itching and biting that comes with trying to catch the pests in canine or feline teeth. Just toss some brewer's yeast into the little guy's food. Evidently, the fleas will be quick to jump ship because they can't stand how the brewer's yeast makes the animal smell. This isn't surprising, since in its pure form, brewer's yeast is a brown, bitter, generally unappetizing substance. But despite its cosmetic drawbacks, it is an excellent source of nutrients such as

- B vitamins for healthy hearts, minds, immune systems, and energy levels
- chromium to help regulate blood sugar
- selenium for antioxidant enhancement
- nucleic acid, to help fight against bacterial and fungal infections

"The therapeutic value of brewer's yeast has been known for years and is appreciated by doctors as a high-quality dietary supplement," says Steven Bailey, N.D., assistant professor at the Northwest Naturopathic College in Portland, Oregon. Brewer's yeast is full of a substance called skin respiratory factor, or SRF, which helps energize the cells involved in mending wounds. SRF is an active ingredient in the well-known hemorrhoid ointment Preparation H. And although we don't advise applying brewer's yeast directly to hemorrhoids, you could put some in your morning smoothie to help speed the healing process.

Another notable thing about brewer's yeast is that it's inexpensive. Anyone watching their pennies can consider using brewer's yeast as a low-cost alternative to buying a cupboard full of vitamins—which can be a pricey prospect. As an added benefit, brewer's yeast also prevents constipation by acting as a bulking laxative, according to Dr. Bailey, an expert in the field of detoxification.

Now that we've discussed nutritional benefits, let's get down to the substance's recreational contribution: As its name suggests, brewer's yeast is most popularly used in the brewing of beer; it is responsible for infusing beer with its distinctive flavor.

The real trick to using brewer's yeast is to disguise its naturally bitter taste by mixing it in with food or drink to make it palatable. Say you find yourself worried that the three-alarm chili you just whipped up is a little too fattening. Toss in some brewer's yeast, and now you can call it healthy. Or if you're making soup or stew and want it to be thicker as well as more nutritious, pour in brewer's yeast to get it to be both. Brewer's yeast also mixes well in tomato juices and smoothies.

Brewer's yeast can be found quite easily in most health food stores and is available in powder, flake, and tablet forms. Because all brands are different, it's best to follow the dosage suggestions on the label.

 ## RECOMMENDED USAGE

There is no RDI for brewer's yeast.

Children
Administer only under the advice of a doctor or health practitioner.

Adults
Powder or Flakes
1–3 teaspoons daily.
Capsules
One 100-milligram capsule up to three times daily.

 CAUTION!

Brewer's yeast is nontoxic and even recommended for pregnant and lactating women because it's such a great source of nutrients. Because of its role as a bulking laxative, however, anyone with intestinal problems may not want to partake or should do so only with professional advice.

An overdose of brewer's yeast may bring on diarrhea and nausea. These symptoms mean stop using it and check with your health practitioner. This shouldn't happen if you restrict yourself to 1 tablespoon per day.

Finally, because of the word *yeast,* some women might worry that brewer's yeast may increase their risk of getting a vaginal yeast infection. Luckily, brewer's yeast has no association with *Candida albicans,* the yeast responsible for those troublesome infections.

BROMELAIN

Overall Rating . . . . *Recommended*

For relieving angina . . . . *Not Recommended*

To treat enlarged prostate . . . . *Not Recommended*

To reduce inflammation . . . . *Recommended*

For preventing blood clots. . . . . *Recommended*

Next time you're packing a bag or backpack to venture out into the wilderness to go on a long hike or bike ride or any other physically demanding trek, consider adding to the aspirin provisions by stuffing some pineapple juice into the bag. Not only will it help with the aches and pains you might feel after a hard workout, but chances are, if you drink pineapple juice as much as you take pain-relieving medications, you'll probably have fewer chances of getting varicose veins and heart attacks. That's because pineapple juice contains bromelain.

Bromelain is an enzyme that helps our bodies absorb all the nutritious things we eat, including vitamins. It's especially adept at breaking down protein so we can reap the nutritious benefits protein has to offer. Studies conducted in Japan and reported in the journal *Medical Science* confirm that bromelain is also an effective anti-inflammatory. Which is why you might be wise to chug down several glasses of pineapple juice after that physically demanding trek you just took or after an accident that may cause swelling and pain.

The reason bromelain is a successful anti-inflammatory is because it promotes the creation of plasmin, which combats swelling. The good news is that drinking pineapple juice or taking bromelain supplements could very well be just as good at reducing swelling and relieving pain as over-the-counter or prescription drugs. Only you won't experience side effects—except maybe a few more trips to the bathroom.

Bromelain works well for other conditions, too. It's excellent at helping to prevent blood clots, which can ultimately lead to stroke and heart attacks, according to a study published in the medical journal *Neurology*. Smokers are particularly at risk for blood clots and would do well to take supplements. Bromelain may also be effective in treating angina (heart pain), enlarged prostate, problems with the pancreas, high blood pressure, tendinitis and bursitis, varicose veins, menstrual cramps, carpal tunnel syndrome, and gout, although studies have been inconclusive.

RECOMMENDED USAGE

There is no RDI for bromelain.

Children
Not advised for children. Administer only under the advice of a doctor or health practitioner.

Adults
Capsules
One 100-milligram capsule up to three times daily.
Tincture
Three drops in an 8-ounce glass of water three times daily.

You can find this botanical wonder in pineapple juice in any grocery store. One 8-ounce glass does the trick. Or your health food store will carry supplements. Try for the kind with labels that read: gelatin digestion unit (GDU) of 450 to 600.

As a potential remedy for carpal tunnel syndrome, take 250 to 500 milligrams per day between meals, in conjunction with vitamin B.

Treat inflammation with 500 milligrams per day.

 CAUTION!

If you experience heart pain or think you have an enlarged prostate, consult a health-care professional for treatment before supplementing. Always mention your intention of taking a supplement to be sure it doesn't interfere with other methods of treatment.

CALCIUM

Overall Rating . . . . *Highly Recommended*

For building strong bones . . . . *Highly Recommended*

For reducing the risk of osteoporosis . . . *Recommended*

For reducing high blood pressure . . . . *Highly Recommended*

For preventing colon cancer . . . . *Not Recommended*

For reducing the symptoms of PMS . . . *Highly Recommended*

It's ironic that the media is saturated with the good news about calcium ("Got milk?"), but our bodies aren't. Calcium is the most prevalent mineral in our bodies, but according to experts, none of us—neither children nor adult women or men—get enough of it. Fact is, next to iron, it's the most deficient mineral in the American woman's diet. Sadly, this results in 25 million post-menopausal, mostly Caucasian or Asian American, women suffering from thin and frail bones, known as osteoporosis. This means 1.5 million broken bones (in both men and women) per year.

Ninety-nine percent of the calcium in our bodies is stored in our bones and teeth—a good place for it since calcium is primarily responsible for building strong bones (which is why it's so critical for children), as well as maintaining them (which is why the rest of us need it).

Bones don't just develop and stay that way forever. Just like skin and hair, they rebuild themselves over and over again. If we start with ample amounts of calcium at a young age, we build bigger and stronger bones to begin with, which, in the end, pays off.

Here's how: By the time you're about thirty-five, you quit making as much of that healthy bone mass and start to rely on the reserves. So, by getting your fill of calcium when you're young, you create a good bone base that you can rely on later. It's a lot like starting an IRA for when you retire: The more you put away, the more you'll have later on to enjoy those golden years.

It's important to keep depositing into that reserve, though, because your bloodstream needs it, too, and will steal it from the reserves in your bones and teeth to maintain the 1 percent necessary for the rest of your body. Kind of a nasty thing to do, but bloodstream calcium is critical for

- regulating heartbeat and maintaining healthy blood pressure
- clotting blood
- transmitting impulses
- contracting muscles
- metabolizing iron and vitamin B_{12}

An August 1998 study in the *American Journal of Obstetrics and Gynecology* found that 1,200 milligrams of calcium helped reduce the symptoms of PMS in 497 women. Researchers at St. Lukes-Roosevelt Hospital Center in New York found the incidence and severity of aches and pains, food cravings, psychological symptoms, and water retention were decreased by as much as 54% with a daily calcium supplement.

Men can also benefit from calcium since it may reduce high blood pressure and prevent colon cancer—conditions more common to men than women. In fact, American epidemiologists have conducted several studies that show a direct relationship between increased calcium supplementation and the reduction of high blood pressure.

The National Osteoporosis Foundation suggests we keep the reserves ample by filling up on three glasses of milk each day. If you're trying to shed a few pounds or if you're lactose intolerant, don't worry! Both fat-free and lactose-free milk have the calcium you need. If you aren't counting calories, keep eating yogurt and cheese—those are the best places to get calcium. You can also find it in proteins such as beans, nuts, tofu, and chickpeas. Salmon and sardines are good sources if you eat them with the bones, while calcium-rich vegetables include kale, spinach, turnip greens, okra, Swiss chard, broccoli, and potatoes. Though calcium works best when vegetables are cooked, try not to ruin the other vitamins in your vegetables by overcooking.

 RDI

Children
400–1,500 milligrams

Adults
25–50 years: 1,000 milligrams
50+ years: 1,000 to 1,500 milligrams

Pregnant and lactating women: 1,200 milligrams

The National Academy of Science urges us not to exceed 2,500 milligrams of calcium per day.

Pregnant and lactating women should increase their calcium intake to 1,200 milligrams. Nursing moms, beware: Your body is doing exactly what a good mother would want it to—making absolutely sure your baby gets enough calcium through your milk. How? By taking it from you, of course. So if you aren't eating enough green leafy vegetables or supplementing efficiently, the baby is stealing it from your bones and teeth. That leaves very little in your reserves and subsequently, a good chance of brittle bones right around the time Junior heads off for college.

While you're enjoying all the goodies that contain calcium, bear in mind that we can't absorb it without adequate amounts of vitamin D. Most commercial milk is fortified with the vitamin for that very reason. But you can also pump up your chances of good absorption by getting thirty minutes of sunshine a day or by eating fortified cereals and other vitamin D–rich foods. It's also good to complement calcium intake with zinc and magnesium. (Check out the sections on vitamin D, zinc, and magnesium in this book to learn more.)

Not everybody enjoys three glasses of milk a day—even if you are rewarded with a milk mustache. And most of us don't eat enough calcium-rich foods to obtain the optimum intake. An easy solution for everyone is to get a supplement.

The best choices are calcium carbonate (it's the most concentrated form, so you get more calcium per tablet than other options), calcium citrate (it's the easiest to absorb and can be found in calcium-enriched juices and other grocery products), calcium gluconate, calcium lactate, and calcium phosphate, which are known to be safe and effective.

Take supplements throughout the day (i.e., 500 milligrams in the morning, 500 milligrams at night) and with a meal. Since your body is busy digesting food, it will allow for more time to absorb the calcium.

It's true that there's a lot of hype about calcium, but the fact is, calcium is important—especially since we don't show signs of deficiencies until it's too late. With that in mind, add this to your list of important things to remember about calcium: Too much caffeine or phosphorous—found in animal proteins and soft drinks—can block calcium from entering your system. That's right—that extra cup of coffee or soda between lunch and dinner could actually be depleting your bone mass! If you're dependent on them, try striking a balance by taking as much calcium as you do phosphorous. This is also true when taking oral contraceptives, antibiotics, and laxatives.

Finally, another sure-fire way to absorb calcium is good old physical exercise. A combination of aerobics and weight lifting, washed down with a little calcium, may slow and even prevent the creeping symptoms of osteoporosis.

 CAUTION!

It has yet to be proven that an excess of calcium causes kidney stones. But if you have kidney stones, stop taking the supplements and see a physician. Calcium supplements are not advised for people who already have kidney disease.

If you take medications for a thyroid condition or high cholesterol, or if you regularly take steroids, antacids, or alcohol, or if you smoke, you are automatically depleting your calcium reserves. Talk with your health care practitioner about how best to compensate.

Hypercalcemia is a very rare condition that has been linked to excessive amounts of vitamin D. Symptoms include constipation, sleepiness, poor appetite, headaches, and general weakness. If you have these symptoms, stop taking calcium supplements and consult with your doctor.

Some people believe calcium supplements cause constipation. Even so, if your only problem is constipation, don't reach for that calcium-blocking laxative! Instead, ease up on the dairy products and calcium supplements, drink a lot of water, and switch to calcium-rich proteins and vegetables that are high in fiber.

Children with calcium deficiencies can get rickets; adults can get osteoporosis, osteomalacia, muscle cramps, and contractions.

CARNITINE

Overall Rating. . . . . *Highly Recommended*

For reducing cholesterol . . . . *Recommended*

When the essential amino acids lysine and methionine get together, they produce carnitine. This nonessential amino keeps the heart and circulatory system in good shape because it

- transports fatty acids into the mitochondria of your heart cells, resulting in energy production
- reduces blood cholesterol
- helps people with coronary artery disease get the most out of limited oxygen, thereby reducing chest pains when exercising

Due to its energizing abilities, carnitine has been used to help people who suffer from chronic fatigue syndrome. Furthermore, studies are currently underway to determine carnitine's potentially beneficial effect in reducing memory loss and mental deterioration in the elderly and people with Alzheimer's. To date, those long-term studies conducted by geriatric facilities nationwide have shown that carnitine helps reduce depression in the elderly.

Carnitine supplements, while not recommended for children, are not known to have any toxic side effects.

 RECOMMENDED USAGE

There is no RDI for carnitine.

Children
Administer only under the advice of a doctor or health practitioner.

Adults
Capsules
One 100-milligram capsule up to three times daily.

AMINO ACIDS

Take away our bones and teeth and what's left? Amino acids (or proteins) in varying combinations. Amino acids are the raw materials used to build our cells and are necessary for life because they regulate our biologic processes by creating enzymes, hormones, and neurotransmitters. The twenty-two amino acids come from our food and, in turn, combine to create over 50,000 different protein molecules that are vital for our bodies to function.

Eight of the amino acids are essential, meaning we need them to survive but can only get them from foods. The remaining fourteen, though equally vital for life, can be made from the essential eight. The essential aminos are isoleucine, leucine, lysine, methionine, phenylalanine, threonine, tryptophan, and valine. The nonessential aminos are alanine, asparagine, aspartic acid, cysteine, glutamic acid, glutamine, glycine, proline, serine, and tyrosine. Four other nonessential aminos—arginine, carnitine, histadine, and taurine—are particularly important for infants and children. In fact, children require higher quantities of protein-rich foods per pound of body weight than adults do.

We get amino acids from our diet. "Complete" proteins are in animal foods such as eggs, meat, fish, and milk. They're complete because they contain all eight of the essential aminos. "Incomplete" proteins are found in plant foods and contain fewer than the essential eight. Plant proteins can be combined, however, to provide the essential aminos needed for optimum health. The National Institutes for Health suggest that, for this purpose, good plant proteins include legumes, soy products, and whole grains. Because running on less than the eight essentials can keep the ones we do have from functioning properly, it's important to get them all into our diets. Amino acids require vitamins B_6, B_{12}, and niacin in order to be metabolized, so be sure to include these vitamins when taking supplements. Also look for supplemental formulas that mirror real proteins so that the much-needed balance of essential and nonessential amino acids—and their correct proportions—are included.

Although the amino acids work together, a number of them have special properties of their own and may therefore be taken individually in supplemental form. These amino acids are described in individual entries. RDIs have not been established for individual amino acids, and recommended doses vary. Therefore, it's best to check with a health practitioner or nutritionist prior to using amino acid supplements to be certain of the correct amount and proper usage.

CAT'S CLAW
(*Uncaria tomentosa*)

Overall Rating . . . . *Highly Recommended*

For alleviating the symptoms of
autoimmune disorders . . . . *Highly Recommended*

When you hear the term "cat's claw" for the first time, you might picture the flexed foot of a fighting feline, claws protruding, poised to attack its victim. A not-too-pleasant picture, especially if the claw is about to break your skin! Keep the fighting image if you must, but put it in this context to more accurately view this amazing herb: The cat's claw attacks an inflamed joint so it no longer creates pain and stiffness in the body. Now, that's a fighter you want on your side.

Grown primarily in the rain forests of the Amazon in Latin America, cat's claw, also known as *una de gato,* is a woody vine that derives its name from two small, sharp thorns at the base of each pair of leaves. Relatively unknown in North America, tea from the inner bark of the stalk and root has been brewed for medicinal purposes in Southern and Central America for centuries.

Only recently have studies in Latin America, Switzerland, Germany, and Italy backed up the anecdotal claims for what this powerful herb can do. Because it contains six oxindole alkaloids, cat's claw effectively stimulates the immune system and increases white blood cell activity, thus helping with immune-deficient illnesses such as AIDS, lupus, fibromyalgia, and chronic fatigue syndrome. Although it cannot be considered a cure for any of these conditions, there is evidence that it can increase the number of T cells we make, justifying its use to boost the immune system.

There's more. Cat's claw contains antioxidant properties and possesses antitumor, antiviral, and anti-inflammatory agents. Given all that, the herb has successfully reduced cancerous tumors and is believed to effectively treat symptoms of arthritis, allergies, rheumatism, gastritis, depression, herpes, and ulcers.

If you're generally healthy and just want to keep your immune system functioning well, supplementing with cat's claw will help. Plus you may even feel more energy along the way.

 ## RECOMMENDED USAGE

There is no RDI for cat's claw. Children should not take this supplement unless supervised by a physician.

Since recent studies show the varied contributions to health this herb offers, most health food stores now carry it.

Adults can take up to 2 grams per day with water at meals. If you are treating serious conditions, such as AIDS, lupus, or cancer, work with a health care professional to determine adequate doses. This is a nontoxic substance, but it's still best to work with a doctor to map out your most effective route to health and to avoid interfering with existing treatments.

 ## CAUTION!

Avoid using cat's claw if you are pregnant or breastfeeding, as it does stimulate the uterus. People on medications for ulcers should not use it, either.

CAYENNE PEPPER
(*Capsicum frutescens*)

Overall Rating . . . . *Highly Recommended*

For treating skin conditions . . . . *Highly Recommended*

"**I** bite!" That's what the botanical name for cayenne pepper means in Greek. And if you've ever bitten into one of these little fiery red devils, you know that the fire is not limited to this tiny pepper's pigment.

Cayenne peppers and other hot chilies, such as jalapeño and habenero peppers, contain capsaicin, a compound that acts as both a furnace and medicine chest. And the hotter the pepper, the more the capsaicin. Cayenne peppers tend to fall in the middle of the heat range—ten times hotter than jalapeños but ten times less hot than habaneros. As you might guess, a little chili pepper goes a very long way.

When you bite into a fresh chili or eat a big forkful of a spicy food, your body immediately reacts by breaking into a sweat. This sweating reaction is beneficial in several ways: speeding up metabolism, increasing blood flow, boosting circulation, and ridding the body of toxins and harmful bacteria.

Besides causing you to sweat and reach for a cold drink, eating cayenne pepper stimulates the production of saliva and gastric juices. While you might think that anything this hot would wreak havoc on your tummy, chili peppers may actually have a soothing effect and may help relieve indigestion and gas. They may even soothe existing ulcers by boosting the production of mucous, helping to protect and heal them.

These natural reactions to cayenne make consuming it useful for people suffering from a variety of ailments, from the common cold to lethargy. But recently, cayenne has revealed an even greater aspect of itself: It travels through our nervous system and triggers the release of something called substance P. No, it's not a vitamin; rather, it's a deterrent against pain. Studies published in *Journal of American Academy of Dermatology* demonstrate that this pain relief is effective both internally and externally—which is why capsaicin is recommended for topical use on painful eczema and psoriasis.

Given what substance P does, you'd think we'd all carry cayenne around in our pockets. Not a bad idea, since substance P literally exhausts our bodies of pain signals. That means if you have a neck pain and apply capsaicin cream to it, after an initial burning sensation, the pain will be alleviated. At the same time, cayenne stimulates the brain to produce endorphins, whose effect compares with that of morphine. This is great news for people combating chronic pain associated with conditions like arthritis, rheumatism, and severe shorter-term illnesses like shingles.

While you consider what your next spicy meal will be, keep this in mind, too. Cayenne exceeds the recommended daily allowance (RDI) of vitamin C and gives us a solid dose of beta-carotene. Beyond providing these two essential nutrients, cayenne is also thought to contribute to

- lowering cholesterol
- protecting against heart disease and stroke
- preventing blood clots

 RECOMMENDED USAGE

There is no RDI for cayenne.

Children
Not advised for children. Administer only under the advice of a doctor or health practitioner.

Adults
Capsules
One 100-milligram capsule up to three times daily.
Tincture
Three drops in an 8-ounce glass of water three times daily.

You can cook delicious meals with the powdered pepper available in any grocery store. Adding up to ½ teaspoon of cayenne pepper to tea or hot water and honey may stimulate your body to act as a decongestant. Drinking cayenne in your tea can also help soothe throat problems such as laryngitis or tonsillitis.

While you may feel warm at first, eating hot spicy food in hot weather or when you have a fever is actually an effective way to cool your body. Your body temperature will drop to compensate for the fire you just stoked inside. If you just can't wait for your body to respond, drinking milk will cool the burning in your mouth. Water, even ice-cold water, probably won't help.

Nasal sprays containing capsaicin are sometimes recommended for migraine headaches.

Capsaicin cream, however, should only be used topically. Apply the cream to painful areas up to four times daily. Use creams with doses of .025 percent to .075 percent capsaicin.

CAUTION!

Contrary to common opinion, cayenne will not cause stomach problems, but taken in very large doses it may damage the liver and kidneys or exacerbate ulcers.

People who suffer from nosebleeds, pregnant women, and nursing mothers may want to limit their consumption of cayenne to culinary uses, if at all.

If you are using fresh chilies, discard the seeds, as they can be toxic, and always remember to wash your hands thoroughly before touching your eyes or any cuts on your body. The same advice goes for over-the-counter ointment.

CERNITIN

Overall Rating . . . . *Highly Recommended*

For reducing enlarged prostate . . . . . . *Highly Recommended*

You may not have heard of cernitin before—most people haven't. No, it's not a vitamin and it's not an herb. Something derived from marine life? Nope. How about a drug? Wrong again. Rather, cernitin is flower pollen extract. But this is nothing to sneeze at. Especially if you're a man over the age of forty and concerned about benign prostatic hyperplasia (BPH), commonly known as an enlarged prostate.

Due to hormonal changes, by the time men are in their fifties, something called dihydrotestosterone prompts the cells in the prostate gland to multiply more than they ought to, which, in effect, enlarges the prostate gland. This is not a particularly dangerous condition, and it *does not* lead to prostate cancer. Symptoms include frequent urination (especially at night), difficulty urinating and interrupted flow, or dribbling during urination. It's uncomfortable, embarrassing, and sometimes painful for millions of men.

Now a little history: Back in the early 1950s over in Sweden, a fellow name Ake Asplund decided that "pollen grain is the source of life to plants," so it must be important to all of us. After extensive research, he was able to extract the digestible parts of plant pollen, get rid of the parts we might be allergic to, and put what's left in a tablet form. By 1959, he realized that this pollen helped relieve prostate problems, specifically by reducing the enlarged prostate gland associated with BPH.

Since then, cernitin has been studied all over the world—in Belgium, China, Great Britain, Germany, Italy, Japan, Poland, Russia, Sweden, and more. The overwhelming evidence from all these studies is that cernitin works to reduce the enlarged gland and, in some cases, even eliminate all prostatic symptoms. One such study conducted in 1993 at the Department of Urology at George-August University in Germany and reported in the *British Journal of Urology* cited a 78 percent improvement rate. A 1996 study conducted in China and reported in *China Medical University* journal claimed a 92 percent improvement rate.

Cernitin is extracted from flower pollen by a specialized process that is critical to its effectiveness. Regular pollen, queen bee pollen, and various other forms of pollen are completely different supplements and have no beneficial effects on the prostate.

Even more good news about cernitin is that it has no side effects, and according to the data gathered from the studies conducted worldwide, it's at least as effective as many prescription drugs such as Hytrin and Proscar.

 ## RECOMMENDED USAGE

There is no RDI for cernitin.

Children
Not for children.

Adult Men
Capsules
Two 63-milligram tablets up to three times daily.

Studies on rats have shown up to 1,000 times the recommended dosage is safe, so increasing the amount of cernitin you take is not a concern, but exceeding the directions on the label is simply a waste of money. Although relatively new to the American market, you should be able to find this product at your health food store.

 CAUTION!

Be sure to work with a health care professional to get a proper diagnosis of BPH before you start using cernitin.

CHAMOMILE

Overall Rating . . . . *Recommended*

For relaxation and as a sleep aid. . . . . *Recommended*

For alleviating menstrual symptoms . . . . *Recommended*

To treat skin conditions . . . . *Recommended*

If life has been a bit hectic of late and you find yourself craving relief from a frazzled mind and twisted nerves, a few quiet moments and a nice cup of chamomile tea may put you at ease. A calming, soothing balm, chamomile also brings relief to insomnia, indigestion, and inflammation.

The Egyptians originally discovered chamomile as a remedy by utilizing two different kinds of plants: Roman chamomile and German chamomile. These plants, virtually identical in both makeup and use, are most commonly known for their ability to calm our buzzing minds, settle our tossing and turning, and help us get to sleep. Some European studies on the use of chamomile as a sleep aid reveal that many people fall into a deep sleep within ten minutes of drinking chamomile tea.

Chamomile is also sipped as a bitter to encourage digestion or to prevent vomiting. It is particularly good for calming a nervous stomach and menstrual cramps—in fact, it was once used to treat the mysterious female malaise known as "the vapors." In the past, chamomile was used to stimulate the uterus and help facilitate labor.

Chamomile is a natural anti-inflammatory. As such, when taken internally, it can help ease discomfort due to back pain and rheumatism. Inhaling chamomile vapor achieves further anti-inflammatory effects by breaking up congestion caused by asthma, hay fever, or bronchitis. In very low doses, it may help provide relief to babies with colic.

Because of their anti-inflammatory and anti-allergy components, chamomile lotions and gels applied to the skin can soothe rashes, insect bites, and eczema and may work as well as, or better than, cortisone, states a now-classic study published in *Herbs, Spices, and Medicinal Plants*. It is also considered safe to use on anal and vulvar irritations.

Chamomile soaps and shampoos are gentle cleansers that don't strip skin or hair of natural oils. Shampoos containing chamomile may also lighten hair color, since chamomile enhances blonde and gold highlights.

You can find chamomile in the form of fresh or dried flowers, ointments, tinctures, essential oils, and homeopathic tablets. It's also available in prepackaged teas, though fresh flowers make the most flavorful brew. Soaps, shampoos, and lotions are available for topical applications.

 RECOMMENDED USAGE

There is no RDI for chamomile.

Children
Administer only under the advice of a doctor or health practitioner.

Adults
Capsules
One 100-milligram capsule up to three times daily.
Extract
Mix 10–20 drops in water up to three times daily.

Tea
Drink one cup daily; you can drink up to three cups if desired.

 CAUTION!

Chamomile flowers look a lot like daisies, because they're members of the same family. If you're allergic to daisies, asters, chrysanthemums, and ragweed, you may also be allergic to chamomile. Using it could cause an irritated, runny, or stuffed-up nose, or sneezing. Topically, allergic reactions could irritate the skin. Those who are allergy prone should not use chamomile.

Drinking a lot of chamomile bitters could cause nausea and vomiting. Chamomile tinctures, used too frequently, also may cause diarrhea. If these symptoms occur, discontinue use.

Finally, pregnant women should avoid using chamomile essential oil internally, as it may stimulate labor.

CHITOSAN

Overall Rating.................. *Highly Recommended*

For weight management.......... *Highly Recommended*

Although some people wouldn't swap a good night's sleep for all the gourmet fare in the world, lots of people around the globe love food. Or use it for comfort. Or depend on it to numb emotions. Or abuse themselves by overeating, under-eating, binge-ing, purging, or addicting themselves. For a variety of reasons, food plays an enormous role not only in our physical well-being, but in our emotional life as well.

Consequently, there are a lot of overweight people around, and yet, this is no simple matter to solve.

Even so, for those people who need a little boost to get started losing weight, who adhere to a relatively good diet and exercise program, and who don't have severe eating disorders, chitosan might be the best choice on the menu.

Chitosan is actually derived from the exoskeletons of shellfish like crab and shrimp. In our bodies, chitosan acts like a super fiber. When it enters the stomach, it turns into a gelatin-like substance that attracts fat molecules to it like a strong magnet. The chitosan itself is insoluble and cannot be absorbed by the body. The fat holds on tightly to the chitosan as it travels through the intestines, and then, along with the chitosan, it is eliminated. And when you don't absorb fat, you don't absorb these calories, which can result in weight loss.

This remarkable phenomenon isn't just another fad created for people hungry to lose weight. It's been studied at prestigious U.S. research centers like Texas A&M University, with successful results reported in the *Journal of the American Medical Association (JAMA)*. It's been researched in Finland, Norway, and Japan, and regardless of the language that reports the news, the results are the same: Chitosan is an effective fat blocker. That means if you eat an occasional candy bar, taking chitosan with it will absorb three to six times the weight of the chitosan in fat, flushing it through the body before it can be absorbed.

In this case, the side effects are nothing but positive. As it blocks the fat, chitosan also

* lowers LDL, or "bad" cholesterol and increases HDL, or "good" cholesterol, thus helping guard against heart disease
* protects against cancer of the colon

These are the direct benefits of using chitosan. But once you start to lose weight, the indirect results can include lowering blood pressure, reducing chances for cancer of the breast and ovaries, decreasing complications or onset of diabetes and gallstones, guarding against gout and kidney stones, helping with back pain and difficulty breathing, relieving symptoms of arthritis, speeding the healing of wounds and broken bones, and acting as an effective antacid.

Don't get too excited, though. You can't use chitosan and its remarkable ability to absorb fat to justify eating gallons of ice cream and cupboards of cookies. It only blocks a finite amount of fat and is not an excuse to overindulge.

Also remember that chitosan doesn't block sugar, it blocks fat. And a lot of the goodies people reach for are packed with sugar. Plus it's most effective for people already eating a low-fat diet who exercise and just want some help getting those extra 10 or 20 pounds off.

RECOMMENDED USAGE

There is no RDI for chitosan.

Children

Not advised for children. Administer only under the advice of a doctor or health practitioner.

Adults

This supplement is available from most health food stores. Adults should take at least 1 gram one-half hour before or with lunch or dinner. Unfortunately, many supplement companies manufacture products that do not contain what they claim. One way to safeguard against purchasing a useless supplement is to purchase one with patent protection, because patent laws require rigorous scientific scrutiny and monitoring. One such patented product containing chitosan is Biozan-C.

Drink at least one 8-ounce glass of water with each tablet or you may get constipated. You should continue drinking plenty of water throughout the day so the fiber in the chitosan doesn't get backed up. Restrict your use of chitosan to no more than 3 grams daily.

 CAUTION!

This is a natural, nontoxic substance. If you have a shellfish allergy, check with a health care professional before taking chitosan, since it is made from the exoskeleton of shellfish. In addition, chitosan will not work if you binge and purge or overeat regularly.

Pregnant or lactating women should not take chitosan. Children under fourteen should also avoid it.

WEIGHT LOSS

Two out of every three Americans are overweight, and one out of three is obese. Unfortunately, these numbers are growing as millions struggle to maintain an ideal body weight.

There is a dizzying array of nutritional supplements that are used for weight loss, including chitosan, chromium picolinate, creatine monohydrate, pyruvate, and St. John's wort. Of these supplements, chitosan shows the most promise.

CHLOROPHYLL

Overall Rating . . . . *Highly Recommended*

For healing wounds . . . . *Highly Recommended*

To treat bad breath . . . . *Highly Recommended*

Next time you're on a meditative saunter in the woods or through a green field, take a moment to reflect on an amazing phenomenon occurring around you. Pick a leaf off a plant or tree and look at it closely. Do you see how the light energy within the green leaf is transforming into chemical energy? That newly formed chemical energy is being stored in bonds of sugar in the leaf. This amazing process of photosynthesis takes place in part because chlorophyll and beta-carotene work together in the membranes of the leaf to absorb light.

And you only thought chlorophyll was good as a breath freshener. But let's face it, anything that contributes to photosynthesis has got to be good for you in other ways, too. According to the *American Journal of Pharmacology,* chlorophyll has positive antibacterial properties as well. Beyond its ability to minimize mouth odor and ward off nasty bacteria, it also contains anti-inflammatory properties. These combined qualities make chlorophyll a good resource for

- healing wounds
- soothing inflamed mucous membranes
- promoting new tissue growth
- reducing opportunities for bacterial infection

- preventing gallstones
- relieving gas and bloating

 RECOMMENDED USAGE

There is no RDI for chlorophyll.

The good news about this well-known, yet taken-for-granted, plant substance is that you can reap its benefits by eating almost anything green, including spinach and parsley. And in any form it contains good amounts of vitamin K.

If you're looking for a supplemental form, it's available in a tablet, powder, or liquid.

To ease digestion and prevent bad breath, take 1 teaspoon or three 100-milligram tablets after each meal. You can take up to 3 teaspoons and nine tablets daily.

 CAUTION!

There are no known side effects. Always read the directions on the label of any product you buy.

CHOLINE

Overall Rating . . . . *Highly Recommended*

To improve mental functioning . . . . . . *Highly Recommended*

To improve liver functioning . . . . *Highly Recommended*

For reducing cholesterol . . . . *Highly Recommended*

For treating bipolar depression . . . . . . *Recommended*

Some days, you may feel that everything you say comes out elegantly and that you should take up the lecture circuit. Other days, you might think it would be better to hide in a closet with duct tape over your mouth. Either way, your brain cells must communicate to each other for you to perceive the message "lecture circuit" or "duct tape." To facilitate this communication, your brain is dependent on choline, a member of the B-complex family, to manufacture a neurotransmitter called acetylcholine. That's the messenger that delivers the news about your emotions and behavior. So choline is the nutrient in charge of making acetylcholine—without which the messages would get mixed up and you'd start to act kind of wacky.

Choline may benefit the brain in other ways, as well. Some doctors use choline—in the form of lecithin—to treat Alzheimer's disease and tardive dyskinesia, a twitching disorder sometimes resulting from the use of antipsychotic medications. Bipolar depression, also known as manic depression, has also shown good results from lethicin supplementation, according to the *American Journal of Psychiatry.* Lethicin has also been thought to help children who are developmentally delayed.

Keeping your brain and nerves on target isn't the only job assigned to choline. It also acts as a personal trainer for your liver: It keeps fats moving so they won't build up. Some studies have indicated that choline may also be helpful for hepatitis, a viral infection of the liver, while in Germany it's regularly used to treat liver damage from alcohol and other toxins; in fact, it's approved by the BDA (the German version of our FDA) for this purpose, based on extensive clinical data. The Germans have also found another effective use for choline: reducing cholesterol.

A little bit of choline is found in most foods, but it's most abundant in lecithin, also known as phyosphatidyl choline. Lecithin helps build the walls of your cells and acts as a natural source of choline. This can be confusing, but to keep it simple, lecithin is also the substance that keeps ice cream and mayonnaise thick!

Animal sources rich in lecithin include caviar, egg yolk, liver, milk, and muscle meats. Good vegetable sources are cabbage, cauliflower, chick peas, green beans, lentils, rice, soybeans, and split peas.

 RDI

Children
Administer only under the advice of a doctor or health practitioner.

Adults
To increase liver functioning: 300–500 milligrams
For lowering cholesterol: 500–800 milligrams

Though RDIs haven't been established for choline, adult men and women should probably get between 100 and 500 milligrams each day. Consult with a health practitioner for individualized advice.

Though supplements are available, the best choice for increasing choline is through lecithin. Not only is it natural, it's also easier for the body to absorb and less irritating than actual choline supplements.

 CAUTION!

Natural choline deficiencies don't exist since we get enough choline in our diets. One exception may be if you take a lot of niacin or nicotonic acid for high cholesterol, because they reduce your ability to absorb choline. If that's the case, you might want to take extra choline.

If you do take a supplement, be aware that very high doses can cause nausea, vomiting, dizziness, and depression. If any of these symptoms show up, stop taking the supplements and contact your health care professional.

Some people have an enzyme deficiency that, in conjunction with large amounts of choline, can make their breath and skin smell fishy. If that's the case, stop taking the choline and the odor will probably go away. Still it would be wise to seek a medical opinion about the possibility of an enzyme deficiency.

CHONDROITIN
AND GLUCOSAMINE

Overall Rating . . . . *Highly Recommended*

For treating symptoms of
osteoarthritis . . . . *Highly Recommended*

There used to be a widely held belief that, as we age, our joints simply wear out. The inevitable and unhappy ending of that scenario is that most people spend their golden years feeling or fighting the pain and being physically restricted by the crippling effects of osteoarthritis. Now, thankfully, we know better, and that grim tale just isn't true.

What is true is that osteoarthritis is a condition in which the body no longer produces enough proteoglycans and collagen, two of the three essential ingredients necessary to give cartilage its resilience and ability to act as a shock absorber. And very often at the same time, certain enzymes are gnawing away at cartilage, contributing to the overall decline of the function of the joint.

The conventional treatment for this pandemic and debilitating condition has been nonsteroidal anti-inflammatory drugs (NSAIDs) such as ibuprofen. They've certainly served their purpose by providing some relief from the pain. But the downside of these drugs is their many unpleasant side effects and the fact that they only respond to the symptoms—not the cause—of the problem.

But there is good news these days. As my coauthors and I wrote in *The Arthritis Cure,* combining glucosamine and chondroitin are now known to halt, reverse, or even cure osteoarthritis.

Just go to the grocery store, pharmacy, or health food store, pick up a pharmaceutical grade of chondroitin sulfate and glucosamine, and you can actually begin treating the cause of the disease at a cellular level and so halt the process of deterioration.

Here's how it works: Healthy cartilage needs three things to stay healthy:

1. water for both lubrication and for carrying the needed nutrients to the cartilage
2. proteoglycans to contain the water
3. collagen to build up the cartilage matrix

As mentioned earlier, osteoarthritis occurs when the body quits making enough proteoglycans and collagen. But if you take chondroitin, it serves as a wrangler, attracting and keeping water in the "pen" with the proteoglycans. It also has the ability to

- act as a shock absorber
- protect cartilage by stopping the enzymes from "chewing" on it
- stimulate production of proteoglycans
- help create glycosaminoglycans (GAGs), which are proteins that bind the water in the cartilage
- work synergistically with glucosamine to protect the old cartilage from premature breakdown while encouraging the synthesis of new cartilage

Glucosamine is the other half of this amazing team. Made up of sugar and amino acids, this busy substance gives structure to cartilage as well as to bones, skin, nails, hair, and other body parts; acts as a building block for the water within cartilage; stimulates the cells that produce GAGs; assists with the production of collagen; normalizes metabolism; and boosts the production of other critical elements within the cartilage mix.

All this adds up to one vital result: Glucosamine helps the body repair damaged or eroded cartilage and therefore, according to a study reported in *Clinical Therapeutics and Current Medical Research,* "it helps reduce pain and restore joint function in people with osteoarthritis."

Studies conducted in the United States and worldwide conclude that chondroitin and glucosamine work simultaneously to brew up new cartilage while warding off those cartilage-eating enzymes. The bottom line is that if you have osteoarthritis, you will most likely experience good or excellent results in rebuilding damaged cartilage by taking this combination of supplements.

The other great news about chondroitin and glucosamine is that taking them produces no side effects. In fact, we already produce them within our bodies to a limited extent. So, unlike NSAIDs, these nontoxic substances settle nicely into their jobs without creating problems for the rest of our system.

 ## RECOMMENDED USAGE

There is no RDI for chondroitin and glucosamine.

Children
Not advised for children. Administer only under the advice of a doctor or health practitioner.

Adults
You do not need a prescription to obtain the supplement, but doses depend on your weight.

	Glucosamine	Chondroitin
Less than 120 pounds:	1,000 milligrams	800 milligrams
120–200 pounds:	1,500 milligrams	1,200 milligrams
More than 200 pounds:	2,000 milligrams	1,600 milligrams

It's best to take the supplement with food and spread out the amount you're taking between two to four doses throughout the day. Also, a number of other supplements help the glucosamine-chondroitin team do its work, acting to catalyze or augment their effectiveness. Among these are vitamins A, C, and E, calcium, magnesium, copper, zinc, boron, chromium, selenium, manganese, and silicon.

To learn more about this whole subject, you may wish to consult *Maximizing the Arthritis Cure* (St. Martin's Press, 1998) or *The Arthritis Cure Cookbook* (Lifeline, 1998).

One final note of praise. The combination of chondroitin and glucosamine can also help dogs, horses, or other animals with arthritic symptoms.

 CAUTION!

Two words of caution:

1. When I was researching and writing *The Arthritis Cure,* I arranged for a laboratory analysis of the many products containing glucosamine and chondroitin to be performed by the University of Maryland at Baltimore. Unfortunately, I found that many brands did not contain both of the active ingredients they claimed, or, if so, they were only in trace quantities.

   On further investigation, it seems the combination of glucosamine and chondroitin is patented by a company called Nutramax, which has licensed it exclusively to Rexall-Sundown. Thus products made by this company and its subsidiaries (Nutramax, Rexall, Sundown, Richardson Labs, and Thompson) all contain the patented product, which is guaranteed to contain the appropriate ingredients. However, all other brands are either violating the patent or are not putting in the proper ingredients, so beware. Your best bet is to stick to products made by the patent holders or their licensees.

2. Although taking these supplements may relieve pain and help rebuild cartilage, your overall health is dependent on eating well, exercising, drinking in moderation, maintaining an ideal body weight, and not smoking. Be careful not to turn to chondroitin and glucosamine to cure all your ills. Only you can do that by being conscious of your habits and maintaining a healthy lifestyle.

ARTHRITIS

Affecting over 35 million Americans, osteoarthritis (OA) is the most common form of arthritis. It is characterized by pain, stiffness, cracking, enlargement, and deformities of the cartilage of an afflicted joint. In advanced stages, inflammation may be present. The joints most commonly affected by OA include the knee, hip, back, neck, and hand joints.

Research has demonstrated that nutritional supplements, namely glucosamine and chondroitin sulfate, and antioxidants (namely vitamins A, C, E, and selenium) can ease or totally alleviate the symptoms of OA, once thought to be a chronic disease controlled only by pain killers.

Glucosamine and chondroitin sulfates—two of the major building blocks of cartilage—are available in supplement form. Studies have shown that glucosamine stimulates the production of cartilage, reduces pain, and improves joint function. Chondroitin sulfates help draw fluids back to the cartilage and also block enzymes that cut off the transport of vital nutrients to the cartilage.

Several forms of glucosamine and chondroitin sulfates are available in health food and drug stores, as well as through mail order. I recommend products that contain both glucosamine and chondroitin. Some products do not deliver what the label says in terms of the amount of the ingredients in the supplements. (See the notes that appear in the Caution! section at the end of the chondroitin and glucosamine entry.)

Also, antioxidants play an important role in preventing the onslaught of free radicals that can further damage cartilage. The most effective antioxidants are "the four ACES"— vitamins A, C, E, and selenium. In addition to controlling tissue damage, these antioxidants can help reduce inflammation and aid the body in assimilating glucosamine and chondroitin sulfates. See individual entries for more information, or you may want to read some of my books on osteoarthritis: *The Arthritis Cure, Maximizing the Arthritis Cure,* and *The Arthritis Cure Cookbook.*

CHROMIUM

Overall Rating................. *Highly Recommended*

For anti-aging properties
(Syndrome X) .... *Highly Recommended*

For regulating blood sugar .... *Highly Recommended*

For weight management.......... *Recommended*

Whether you've just run the Boston Marathon or put in an extra long day at work, chromium is what helped maintain your energy. That's because it's an essential mineral for producing insulin, the hormone that regulates how much sugar is in our blood. Blood sugar—or glucose—is the fuel we burn for energy.

People with overly high blood sugar levels have diabetes, while in hypoglycemics, these levels are too low. Insulin keeps the body from these extremes by moving glucose out of the blood and into the cells, where it can be utilized or kept until we need it.

Trivalent chromium's relation to insulin production can also affect cholesterol. Too little chromium can mean not enough insulin, which leads to poor use of blood sugar. When this happens, the body uses fats, instead of glucose, for energy. Consequently, there's a reserve of cholesterol left in the blood, creating a veritable garbage dump in the arteries.

Scientists have discovered other links between chromium and insulin sensitivity. Specifically, researchers have concluded that four of the underlying diseases associated with aging are all part of one syndrome, called Syndrome X. The key to understanding, diagnosing, and treating Syndrome X, researchers believe, is how the body processes insulin, and the first sign of diabetes (or insulin resistance) usually indicates the presence of the syndrome's three other conditions, namely obesity, high blood pressure, and high cholesterol. According to studies in *Nutrition,* the *Western Journal of Medicine,* and the *Journal of Nutrition,* an effective way to combat Syndrome X is to take chromium, specifically niacin-bound chromium or chromium polynicotinate.

In addition to regulating your blood sugar and cholesterol—without the side effects of medications—chromium may also improve muscle tone and burn fat, according to studies published in *Sports Medicine.* In fact, studies conducted on male athletes showed an increased capacity to build muscle tissue when supplementing with chromium. This indirectly led to fat loss, since greater muscle mass leads to greater fat burning. Some research even suggests that chromium may increase longevity.

Beer connoisseurs will be glad to know their favorite brew is a great source of chromium, thanks to one of its main ingredients: brewer's yeast. Other foods abundant in chromium include beef, cheese, chicken, clams, and liver. Plant and vegetable sources include broccoli, corn oil, grape juice, molasses, potatoes (with the skin), wheat germ, and whole-grain breads and cereals.

 ## RECOMMENDED USAGE

There is no RDI for chromium.

Children
Administer only under the advice of a doctor or health practitioner.

Adults
25–50 years: 50–200 micrograms
50+ years: 50–400 micrograms

People who eat a lot of refined grains (and let's face it, most of us do), may be a little low on chromium since whole grains lose three quarters of their chromium when refined. Getting a lot of strenuous exercise, particularly running, may also deplete chromium reserves due to the energy demands it makes on the body. The same is true for pregnancy. Finally, as we get older, our body won't retain chromium the way it used to.

 CAUTION!

The effects of chromium supplementation are most dramatic in people with diabetes or hypoglycemia. If you have one of these conditions, speak with your doctor about a chromium supplement to help control blood sugar.

When in search of a good chromium supplement, choose either chromium picolinate niacin-bound chromium (also known as chromium polynicotinate), or glucose tolerance factor.

In its dietary form, trivalent chromium is not known to be toxic at any dosage.

ANTIAGING

Of course, aging cannot be cured, but it *can* be slowed. The latest thinking is that aging is largely a combination of four conditions: excess weight, a poor cholesterol balance, heightened blood pressure (called hypertension when it gets too high), and insulin resistance (leading to diabetes). Together these add up to an overall condition called Syndrome X.

Fortunately, Syndrome X can be slowed and even reversed by a combination of supplements, the most important of which is chromium, best taken in the form of chromium polynicotinate.

COD LIVER OIL

Overall Rating. . . . . *Highly Recommended*

For fighting cancer. . . . . *Highly Recommended*

To prevent clogged arteries. . . . . *Highly Recommended*

To lower high blood pressure . . . . *Highly Recommended*

To relieve the symptoms of
rheumatoid arthritis. . . . . *Highly Recommended*

To reduce cholesterol . . . . *Highly Recommended*

Ask any parent—or grandparent—today about cod liver oil and they'll just squirm. That's because our foremothers knew a lot more than we once gave them credit for. And despite the taste, cod liver oil really provides your body with protection against the elements. That's because it contains EPA and DHA, or omega-3 essential fatty acids, which can

- strengthen cell membranes, blocking cancer from the nutrients it needs to form tumors
- thin blood and prevent clogged arteries
- lower high blood pressure
- relieve the swelling and stiffness caused by rheumatoid arthritis, without the side effects of medication
- reduce blood cholesterol when taken in conjunction with a low-fat diet

Cod liver oil does a lot to keep the heart healthy. Like many fish oils, it prevents blood platelets—which are what form blood clots—from building up in arteries. Ultimately, then, it is thought to reduce the risk of heart attack. In fact, population studies have shown that cod liver oil (an omega-3 oil) significantly reduces the risk of developing heart disease at all and can actually reverse some of the damage for those who've already had problems with their hearts! And a few dozen double-blind studies have come up with the same finding: fish oil supplements are effective in reducing blood pressure.

Fortunately, it's easy to get enough of this form of omega-3 fatty acid. Just help yourself to some fresh cod, mackerel, tuna, or salmon (avoid the deep-fried kind that comes with chips slathered in grease). Or buy supplements. Beware, however, that if you choose oil or capsule supplements, they should contain vitamin E because it prevents the oil from turning rancid. (It's a good idea to take an E supplement along with any form of cod liver oil, since it prevents the oil from oxidizing in the body.)

Some people complain of fish breath when they take cod liver supplements—a rather rude side effect. Time release capsules will keep that fishy smell at bay, keeping your breath kissably fresh.

 ## RECOMMENDED USAGE

There is no RDI for cod liver oil.

Children
Administer only under the advice of a doctor or health practitioner.

Adults
Capsules
One capsule up to three times daily.
Liquid
One or two tablespoons daily.

CAUTION!

Like all fish oils, cod liver oil thins the blood. Supplementation, then, may cause a delay in the blood's ability to clot—though not any more than taking aspirin for its blood-thinning benefits. Just the same, people with blood-clotting troubles or those on blood-thinning drugs should avoid cod liver oil supplementation.

Cod liver oil won't significantly lower cholesterol in people who eat diets high in saturated fat. In fact, adding cod liver oil to a high-fat diet could actually *increase* cholesterol levels. Fish oil only helps lower cholesterol in conjunction with a low-fat diet.

Diabetics should refrain from taking any kind of fish oil supplement, including cod liver oil, because it may increase blood sugar levels.

Cod liver oil is high in vitamins A and D, and too much of either of those vitamins can be toxic.

COENZYME Q-10

Overall Rating. . . . . *Highly Recommended*

To treat heart conditions . . . . *Highly Recommended*

For boosting the immune system. . . . . *Highly Recommended*

Most days find us occupied with daily life, so we often forget that even amidst our most mundane activities, the synergistic organism that is our body is accomplishing mind-boggling feats. We have so many interlinking moving parts, each relying on a number of others to function, that it's a good thing our bodily processes are automatic; can you imagine if we had to remember all this? Take the functions of coenzyme Q-10 (CoQ10), for example.

Each of our cells has a mini energy center called the mitochondrion, which produces adenosine triphosphate (ATP), the energy the body uses to function. CoQ10 regulates the electrical currents in the mitochondria, which enables them to function. The system is similar to a string of lights—if the CoQ10 bulb goes out, none of the others will work. The ultimate result is that CoQ10 helps maintain energy. Anyone feeling run down from a hectic schedule or a recent illness may benefit from it. In fact, it's often recommended for the elderly and people who have chronic fatigue syndrome. It may also help increase endurance during exercise.

CoQ10 is found everywhere in the body, but it's most concentrated and makes some of its greatest contributions in the heart. Although it's still considered a nutritional supplement in the United States, doctors in Japan have been prescribing CoQ10 as a treatment for heart failure since the mid 1970s. CoQ10 keeps hearts healthy by

- relieving angina
- preventing congestive heart failure
- lowering blood cholesterol
- normalizing irregular heartbeat
- treating mitral-valve prolapse
- possibly lowering blood pressure and normalizing blood sugar

That's enough to make anyone smile, but CoQ10 can even make that smile prettier. Gum disease, or gingivitis, may actually be reversed by supplemental CoQ10. Of course, just using the supplement won't be enough—you'll still need to brush and floss.

And if all of this isn't enough, CoQ10 is a fabulous antioxidant. Some research shows that its ability to wipe out free radicals could minimize or halt tumor growth, especially breast cancer. Taken over a period of time, CoQ10 may also help the immune system fight infections, reports *The Journal of Experimental Medicine.*

We manufacture CoQ10 in our bodies, but it's also found in fishy foods, like mackerel, tuna, and sardines, and in proteins such as beef, organ meats, peanuts, and tofu. Rice bran, spinach, vegetable oils, and wheat germ also contain CoQ10. Beware, however, that cooking and processing foods pretty much destroys this valuable coenzyme, so you're better off taking a supplement if you think you're not getting enough.

 ## RECOMMENDED USAGE

There is no RDI for CoQ10.

Children

Administer only under the advice of a doctor or health practitioner.

Adults

CoQ10 is getting increased attention in Western medicine, but RDIs and symptoms of deficiency remain undefined. A daily dose of 30 to 60 milligrams of CoQ10 up to three times per day should give good results, though people have taken up to 200 milligrams without any problems. Individuals taking CoQ10 for their heart may take up to 300 milligrams per day under a doctor's supervision.

A variety of CoQ10 supplements are easy to find in any local health food store. Taking the supplement in the form of gel capsules may be the best bet—not only are these easy for the body to absorb, they're also easy to swallow.

 CAUTION!

Most nutritional experts have found CoQ10 to be very safe. However, extremely high amounts of CoQ10 could upset your stomach or give you diarrhea. In that case, stop taking the supplements and contact your health care practitioner.

COPPER

Overall Rating . . . . *Highly Recommended*

To improve heart function . . . . *Highly Recommended*

For relieving symptoms of arthritis
(taken transdermally) . . . . *Recommended*

Reach the top of a steep hiking trail or the surface of a pool after having traversed its full length under water, and you'll want nothing more than to fill your lungs with air. And though it's often said that breath is life, few of us realize that without the copper reserves in our body, we'd be deprived of this life-sustaining faculty.

Copper is a mineral with many responsibilities, but its first priority is respiration. It helps us breathe by regulating the absorption and release of iron. Iron, in turn, is essential for the formation of hemoglobin, the protein that infuses our red blood cells with oxygen. Because copper helps us employ iron, one of its benefits is the resulting increase in energy. Our bodies also require copper for a number of other purposes, including

- production of a blood antioxidant we make in-house, called superoxide dismutase
- formation of healthy red blood cells and the flexibility that enables blood vessels and arteries to literally "go with the flow"
- construction of the protective membranes that fit over our nerves

Additionally, copper is responsible for manufacturing the proteins collagen and elastin, which keep bones, cartilage, skin, tendons, blood vessels, and lungs sturdy and elastic, as needed; making melanin, the pigment that colors skin and hair; and possibly lowering cholesterol.

Due to copper's association with building and repairing tissue, arthritis sufferers often use copper bracelets. Doctors are skeptical about whether or not this works, but a double-blind study conducted in Australia indicated that, in fact, it does. However, one study does not a definitive endorsement make, and the likelihood of gaining substantial mineral intake from a bracelet needs much more research.

Copper may be mined from many foods, but you can also get it from your water if you have copper pipes or from cooking with copper pots and pans. The most abundant source of copper is seafood, particularly cod, crab, lobster, mussels, oysters, salmon, shrimp, and the little-known whelk. Copper is also plentiful in nuts, whole grains, legumes, raisins, and liver. Because processing destroys the copper found in most foods, the typical American diet isn't as rich in copper as was originally thought.

 RDI

Children
.4–2.5 milligrams

Adults
25–50 years: 3 milligrams
50+ years: 3 milligrams

When using a copper supplement, nutritionists advise taking it in a 1 to 10 ratio with zinc. That's because zinc and copper are in competition with each other for your body's attention. So when taking the recommended 3 milligrams of copper, be sure to also take 30 milligrams of zinc.

 CAUTION!

Having a copper deficiency is rather uncommon and tends to affect people who are severely malnourished. Deficiencies have been known to occur in babies who drink only cow's milk, which is low in copper. As a result, they may have diarrhea and look very pale. Pregnant women are also sometimes copper deficient.

The type of mild copper deficiency most common to the average person would include symptoms of anemia, high cholesterol, low white blood count, and the sensation that nothing tastes good.

Except for people who have the rare hereditary condition known as Wilson's disease, copper has no toxic effects. However, too much copper will lower zinc levels (they compete with each other), and low zinc can cause you to lose sleep, be depressed, and even make your hair fall out. In women, it may also result in irregular menses. For these reasons, it's very important to keep that 10 to 1 zinc-copper ratio in mind—and in practice.

CRANBERRY

Overall Rating. . . . . *Highly Recommended*

For treating bladder infection
(cystitis). . . . . *Highly Recommended*

We all know that vitamin C is good for us. It's an important antioxidant. It helps boost the immune system. And it's found in a variety of different foods. But for some reason, most of us limit our conscious intake of vitamin C to either supplements or brightly colored citrus fruits like oranges and grapefruits. And yet, there are so many other "colorful" places to find a good shot of C—especially when you consider that the delicious red cranberry is chock-full of this precious vitamin, and when eaten whole or drunk as juice, it can provide you and your diet with a real pick-me-up.

First documented in a classic 1962 study in the *Wisconsin Medical Journal* (and verified myriad times since), cranberry juice is also a widely used and effective treatment for cystitis, or urinary tract infection. That's because cranberries contain a compound that basically prevents bacteria from attaching itself to the walls of the urinary tract. So, if you are experiencing burning and irritation while urinating, blaze over to the health food store and purchase a bottle of natural, unsweetened cranberry juice (the juice at the grocery story is packed with sugar, which will irritate the condition). Drink several glasses a day until the symptoms subside.

Cranberries also act as a natural diuretic and antibiotic. Drinking several glasses of (again, natural) juice (or taking concentrated cranberry tablets) each day can offer real relief, especially if you are prone to recurring infections.

Because of their high vitamin C content, cranberries may also provide protection against cancer, heart disease, high blood pressure, infertility, eye damage and deterioration, and the common cold.

 RECOMMENDED USAGE

There is no RDI for cranberries.

Children
Not advised for children at therapeutic levels. Administer only under the advice of a doctor or health practitioner.

Adults
Capsules
One 1-gram capsule up to three times daily.
Juice
Drink three to five glasses (8 ounce) daily until symptoms subside. Make sure to drink an equal amount of water.

 CAUTION!

Urinary tract infections can be dangerous—especially if you're pregnant. If you have an active infection, visit a health practitioner to determine the best course of treatment.

CREATINE

Overall Rating . . . . *Not Recommended*

For building lean muscle . . . . *Not Recommended*

For burning fat . . . . *Not Recommended*

Actually intended for athletes, creatine monohydrate reportedly enhances the strength, intensity, and endurance of athletic functions requiring short periods of intense exercise. That's why it's the newest craze for bodybuilders.

Creatine is a naturally occurring chemical that's stored in muscles and fuels the muscle's ability to contract, especially for concentrated, short-term purposes. Taking creatine supplements may quicken the time it takes for muscle contraction to happen. It might also rapidly build up muscles for a short period of time.

If you're a competitive cyclist, football or basketball player, short-distance swimmer, weight lifter, or other committed athlete who needs an extra "bump" to make that split-second difference in timing or to press that extra pound, creatine might be of help to you. But be mindful that it supplies energy blasts for on average between six and eight seconds, although it can go up to thirty seconds. It's also important to keep in mind that the energy blast tends to occur at the early stage of the activity, when you may need it the least. If you already have high levels of creatine in your muscles, it won't help at all. The jury is still out on this supplement. While many people have reported great results from creatine supplementation, controlled studies show less-than-favorable results.

RECOMMENDED USAGE

There is no RDI for creatine, but you can consume it by eating steak or fish or by drinking milk. Vegetarian athletes who need that intense, short-term burst may benefit more than meat-eating athletes.

Children
Not advised for children. Administer only under the advice of a doctor or health practitioner.

Adults
If you decide to give creatine a try, you can choose from a powder, capsule, candy, or gum form. For greatest effectiveness, try taking 5 grams four times per day for up to six days. After that, reduce the amount to 2 to 5 grams per day. While supplementing with creatine, be sure to drink 2 quarts of water per day to avoid dehydration. And although the label might instruct you to take it with fruit juice, it's best with water.

 CAUTION!

Creatine is not good for endurance athletes because it somehow interferes with the body's mechanism to sweat. Therefore, there is danger of dehydration.

If you experience muscle cramps, spasms, strains, or pulls, discontinue use and consult a health care practitioner. Don't take large doses for more than six days at a time.

There is some question about whether using creatine supplements may interfere with the body's ability to manufacture its own creatine. *Use this substance at your own risk.*

CYSTEINE

Overall Rating. . . . . *Recommended*

To block harmful free radicals . . . . *Recommended*

There are only three amino acids that contain sulfur: cysteine, methionine, and taurine. Cysteine, in particular, emits a form of sulfuric acid that blocks free radicals. It also helps us make glutathione, the most prevalent antioxidant in the body. Cysteine and glutathione team up in the liver, where they gather and dispose of harmful toxins. Some of these toxins include free radicals set loose by everyday pollutants, cigarette smoke, alcohol consumption, and harmful metals.

 RECOMMENDED USAGE

There is no RDI for cysteine.

Children
Administer only under the advice of a doctor or health practitioner.

Adults
Capsules
One 100-milligram capsule up to three times daily.

CAUTION!

Cysteine may affect insulin levels. Diabetics, therefore, are not advised to use cysteine supplements without seeking the advice of a health practitioner.

DANDELION
(*Taraxacum officinale*)

Overall Rating . . . . *Recommended*

To improve liver functioning . . . . *Recommended*

If you do yard work, you might have a love-hate relationship with the dandelion. An immaculate lawn requires you to dig it, poison it, or chop it down. But dandelion, with its bright yellow, sunny flowers and puffballs of seeds, is one of those plants that reminds us of childhood. Who can resist plucking a dandelion and blowing the seeds into the wind? Go ahead. Alternate the years in which you spare the dandelion and slay it. That way, the neighbors won't get too upset and you can have some childhood fun, too.

Plus you never know when a little dandelion might come in handy. It is an incredibly useful plant, which we would probably cultivate if we weren't trying to keep up with the Jonses—or if we knew how to use it.

Believe it or not, some people think dandelions actually taste good and eat them much like lettuce and other greens. Young, tender dandelion leaves can be added to salads, cooked like spinach, and puréed into juice. Ever had dandelion wine? That's made from distilled blossoms. Dandelion roots can also be roasted, ground, and drunk like coffee. Add a little ground, roasted burdock root to this concoction, and you have a traditional remedy for arthritis. Which leads us to its medicinal properties.

The entire dandelion plant is full of helpful vitamins and minerals. We're often told to eat carrots to strengthen our eyes, but drinking a tea made from dandelion flowers will actually provide even more vitamin A than carrots will. Dandelion is also full of potassium.

Tea made of dandelion roots and leaves can stimulate the liver and gallbladder and may help with symptoms of cirrhosis, hepatitis, gallstones, and jaundice, according to David Hoffman, author of *The New Holistic Herbal*. In tea form, it's also a strong natural diuretic, recommended to relieve swelling and water retention. In any form, dandelion will fill you up with iron, beta-carotene, and vitamin C, making it helpful in fighting anemia and generally strengthening your body.

If you're still not convinced that you'd be better off eating, rather than exterminating, this plant, here are more good things dandelions may do:

- stimulate digestion
- ease constipation
- fight infections such as measles, chicken pox, pneumonia, bronchitis, and poison ivy
- break a fever
- cleanse the body of toxins
- fight hypertension
- strengthen the heart
- lower cholesterol levels
- increase milk supply in nursing mothers

If eating the plant doesn't make your mouth water, consider other medicinal applications. Try a poultice of crushed dandelions to help soothe boils and abscesses. Add dandelion leaves to your bath or use it to steam your face as a general tonic. And if you've ever thought about making natural dyes or paints, dandelion flowers produce an excellent yellow color, while the whole plant can be used to make—surprise!—magenta.

RECOMMENDED USAGE

There is no RDI for dandelion.

Children
Not advised for children. Administer only under the advice of a doctor or health practitioner.

Adults
Capsules
One 100-milligram capsule up to three times daily.
Fluid Extract
One to two teaspoons in an 8-ounce glass of water three times daily.

For a diuretic, take up to 20 milligrams of puréed leaves as a juice.

To cleanse the body of toxins or stimulate the liver, take 4 to 6 teaspoons daily. The decoction is best, however, if you're cleaning the liver. You can drink at least three cups per day for six months.

 ## CAUTION!

Dandelion is generally a very safe plant. However, if you gather dandelions, make sure they have not been sprayed with any dangerous chemicals. And gather them when they are young, since the leaves become bitter with age.

Dandelion sap can be corrosive, so if you are using it topically, be careful to apply it only where you need it. Those with kidney disease should use with caution because of the high potassium content.

DEVIL'S CLAW
(*Harpagophytum procumbens*)

Overall Rating . . . . *Highly Recommended*

To reduce inflammation . . . . *Highly Recommended*

To lower cholesterol. . . . . *Highly Recommended*

You've probably read something about the healing power of the human touch and the therapeutic power we may be able to spread through our hands. But who in their right mind would think claws would be of any use in healing, especially the healing of bodily aches and pains? Well, as improbable as it sounds, a thorny, painful-looking tuber from Namibia called devil's claw may be an effective anti-inflammatory. Although a study published in *The Canadian Medical Association Journal* claims that results are inconsistent, some people did find devil's claw greatly relieved symptoms of

- osteoarthritis
- gout
- lumbago (back pain)
- sciatica
- rheumatism

Another study published in *The Handbook of Medicinal Herbs*, however, states there is firm, conclusive evidence that devil's claw can help lower levels of serum cholesterol and uric acid. That's good news for people with gout. Devil's claw may also work as a diuretic, a sedative, and a mild pain reliever.

RECOMMENDED USAGE

There is no RDI for devil's claw.

Children
Not advised for children. Administer only under the advice of a doctor or health practitioner.

Adults
To relieve symptoms of osteoarthritis, take 1 to 3 grams in capsule form per day. When acute symptoms diminish, reduce the amount to 15 milliliters of tincture per day. Look for devil's claw in combination with angelica, St. John's wort, bogbean, white willow bark, or celery seed.

If you prefer a decoction, take a teaspoon of devil's claw in water twice daily.

 ## CAUTION!

Devil's claw may increase stomach acid and irritate existing ulcers. Do not take devil's claw if you are pregnant.

DHEA

Overall Rating . . . . *Not Recommended*

To reduce the likelihood of heart disease. . *Not Recommended*

To reduce the likelihood of cancers . . . . *Not Recommended*

For relieving symptoms of lupus . . . . . . *Recommended*

To increase libido in
menopausal women. . . . . *Recommended*

The quest for eternal youth has for centuries captured the imagination. And though none of us would want to sacrifice the wisdom and experience that only growing older can bring, let's face it—we have a universal desire to age with grace. So prick up your ears: DHEA (dehydroepiandrosterone) may help make that wish a reality.

What is DHEA? Most folks think of it as a nutritional supplement, but in truth it's a steroid hormone secreted by the adrenal glands. Once the adrenals set it loose, DHEA travels to the liver, where it's transformed into male and female hormones. Over time, our bodies make less and less DHEA—by middle age we have only half of the DHEA we had in our twenties—and it continues to drop for the rest of our lives. As a result, researchers think that increasing DHEA levels in people over the age of forty will help reduce—and even reverse—a number of aging problems, such as

- susceptibility to illness
- poor memory
- diabetes

- low energy
- depression
- muscle loss

Although DHEA won't make us live longer, it may very well improve the overall quality of life in later years.

Studies have shown that DHEA may also fight cancer by producing natural killer cells that attack cancer cells before they can take root. Men with heart disease may also benefit from DHEA, as it seems to create a blood-thinning effect, while women with the rare and serious illness lupus have been able to reduce their medication by increasing their DHEA levels, according to a double-blind study conducted at Queens University in Northern Ireland.

One application that has proven to be an effective use of DHEA is the treatment of decreased sex drive in postmenopausal women. Because of the hormone's similarity to testosterone, it is thought to increase the libido with no overriding side effects, says Christiane Northrup, M.D., author of *Women's Bodies, Women's Wisdom*. The dosage, starting at about 5 milligrams per day orally, should be regulated by your doctor or health care practitioner.

 ## RECOMMENDED USAGE

There is no RDI for DHEA.

Children

Administer only under the advice of a doctor or health practitioner.

Adults

To date, there are neither RDIs nor deficiency symptoms for DHEA. Although many substances created in the body are also found in different foods, DHEA is an original. The obscure Mexican wild yam has been rumored to have some DHEA, but otherwise no other foods are known to contain it.

DHEA supplements are available in the form of capsules, liquids, sprays, and tablets. Capsules tend to be easier to digest, while the liquids and sprays call for a lower dosage.

 CAUTION!

DHEA supplements are easily found on the shelves of neighborhood pharmacies and health food stores. Most nutritionists agree, however, that it's best to take DHEA only under professional medical supervision. That's because DHEA supplements are intended to create a normal level of this hormone in the body, not a surplus. So if you're under the age of forty, don't take DHEA supplements—your body already makes enough.

DHEA is not known to have any serious short-term side effects, but long-term effects are unknown and could be serious, such as promoting tumor growth. Exceeding normal levels may stimulate the liver to produce male and female hormones that aren't needed. An excess of male hormones (called androgens), could result in androgen-related side effects, including oily skin, mood swings, a deeper voice, prostate cancer, and increased hair growth. These will go away once the DHEA supplements are stopped, but if you experience such symptoms, be sure to see your health care provider to ensure that your hormones remain in healthy balance.

DONG QUAI
(*Angelica sinensis*)

Overall Rating . . . . *Recommended*

For relieving pain . . . . *Recommended*

To treat gynecological conditions . . . . *Recommended*

When women learn about all the things dong quai can do, it could tempt them to fire their doctor, then dash to the medicine cabinet and trash all the drugs they've tried for treating menstrual cramps, menopause, constipation, and general pain. So, at this moment, if you're a woman and feeling the downside of PMS, or if you're cramping up right now, just take a deep breath, relax, and be grateful that there are alternatives available to you.

Used in Chinese medicine for thousands of years to treat most gynecological conditions, dong quai has earned the nickname "empress of herbs." Such an elegant name might lead you to believe that it's a flower from this herb that contains the remedies for female difficulties, but it's actually the root that provides its broad medicinal properties.

Known as a blood purifier, dong quai can effectively regulate periods, especially for women who have recently stopped taking oral contraceptives. It has also been successful at alleviating symptoms of PMS, as well as menstrual cramps. As a uterine stimulant, it's not advised during pregnancy, but immediately after the baby is born, it's an excellent remedy to help stabilize the uterus.

Menopausal women experiencing hot flashes, vaginal dryness, and debilitating fatigue may also find relief from the organic estrogen-producing properties of the herb. Some menopausal women have found themselves symptom-free after using both dong quai and wild yam, nature's plant source for progesterone. Given that the hormonal properties in these plants can either help protect deterioration of bones or help build new ones, dong quai may also be effective in combating osteoporosis.

Men shouldn't feel left out, however. According to the well-respected Japanese medical journal *Yakuga Zassh,* "dong quai is 1.7 times stronger than aspirin to relieve mild pain." So, if you're hurting for one reason or another, take a capsule of dong quai and avoid those acidic side effects of aspirin. But as yet no solid evidence exists.

There's more! Dong quai is thought to be useful in treating symptoms of rheumatism, hypertension, anemia, high blood pressure, neuralgia, heart pain, arthritis pain, blurred vision, palpitations, and even constipation. But as yet no solid evidence exists.

In China and Taiwan, doctors inject dong quai in strategic acupuncture points to ease angina and arthritis. In Asia, it is also recommended for stimulating the liver.

 ## RECOMMENDED USAGE

There is no RDI for dong quai.

Children
Not advised for children. Administer only under the advice of a doctor or health practitioner.

Adults
You can find this popular herb in the form of powder, tea, or the root itself, in almost any health food store.

To treat menopausal symptoms, take up to 500 milligrams per day.

To make a decoction, combine 30 grams of the powder with 500 milliliters of water. Take it in three doses.

To make tea, combine 2 teaspoons of the grated root in 1½ pints of water. Cover and simmer twenty minutes. Drink 1 cup per day for general pains or to strengthen your liver.

 CAUTION!

Since dong quai is a powerful herb that contains hormones, consult a health-care professional before using it. And as it affects both the blood and uterus, don't use it at any time during pregnancy.

It's also not advised if you are a heavy bleeder during your period, if you have blood-clotting problems, or if you experience nosebleeds. Avoid it as well if you have a fever, diarrhea, a distended abdomen, a sore throat, or any kind of tumor growth on any female reproductive organ.

MENOPAUSE

Women entering menopause are besieged by several discomforting symptoms—hot flashes, mood swings, headaches, vaginal drying, fatigue, and irritability—due in large part to the drop in estrogen levels. Although most of these symptoms eventually disappear, they do, nevertheless, create great unpleasantness.

Although no nutritional supplement has been found to be more effective than the pharmaceutical alternatives, supplements are a useful weapon in helping to combat many of these symptoms.

The most widely used and recommended supplements and natural remedies include dong quai, flaxseed oil, ginseng, lysine, magnesium, royal jelly, and soy. (See the individual entries for recommendations, indications, and efficacy ratings.)

ECHINACEA

Overall Rating . . . . *Highly Recommended*

For treating bacterial and
viral infections . . . . *Highly Recommended*

To strengthen the immune system . . . . *Highly Recommended*

For healing wounds (topically) . . . . . . *Highly Recommended*

The Thanksgiving story we're usually told begins with the *Mayflower*, gets into how the Native Americans taught the Pilgrims how to use corn, and somehow ends with pumpkin pie. Another version could begin with how the Plains Indians used the root of the coneflower—or echinacea—to doctor snakebites, toothaches, and wounds. It could then lead into how the Native Americans introduced this herb to the settlers and end with how the settlers adapted echinacea to their own lifestyles to relieve the symptoms of colds and flu.

Echinacea, among the best known and most popular herbal remedies, is used to

* combat bacterial and viral infections, including colds and flu
* strengthen the immune system
* help heal skin wounds and irritations

The chief use for echinacea is to ward off viral and bacterial infections like colds, influenza, urinary tract infections, and kidney infections. In some cases, it may even ease the aftereffects of food poisoning.

There are a couple of very good reasons for echinacea's success. Between each of our cells is a natural barrier that separates our healthy tissues from disease-causing organisms. The chief culprit in destroying this barrier is an enzyme known as hyaluronidase. Because echinacea has been shown to prevent this enzyme from forming, it helps the body fight off viruses and other infections, according to a German study published in *Arznehim Forsch*.

Echinacea is thought to keep up our immune defense also because it contains a polysaccharide that intensifies macrophages. Macrophages are a kind of killer cell that protects us against all sorts of pathogens—including cancer. According to a recent National Cancer Institute study, by strengthening these macrophages, it's thought that echinacea may actually prevent malignant tumors from growing.

Snakebites and arrow punctures were frequent maladies in the time of the Plains Indian but are of little concern today. And although echinacea is primarily used for bacterial and viral infections, it's also useful as a topical treatment for fungal infections, eczema, psoriasis, scrapes, and insect bites. Not only will it take the sting and itch out of a bug bite, it's really good for killing bugs, too.

Treat skin conditions with the powder by giving the afflicted area a good dusting. Infected wounds, however, should be washed with diluted tincture. Apply creams containing echinacea directly to fungal infections or psoriasis and eczema.

 ## RECOMMENDED USAGE

There is no RDI for echinacea.

Children
Administer only under the advice of a doctor or health practitioner.

Adults

For symptoms of flu, kidney, and urinary tract infections, drink up to 5 milliliters of the tincture at full strength, every couple of hours. Swallowing capsules is another good way to treat these symptoms. Morning, noon, and night, take an average of 800 milligrams (two 400-milligram capsules) when you first feel sick. As an immune booster, echinacea is often combined with another popular herb, goldenseal. Gargle with 10 milliliters of the tincture in a glass of warm water to take the sting out of a sore throat.

Use topical echinacea cream for relief as needed.

 CAUTION!

Echinacea is nontoxic, but large amounts can cause stomach upset and dizziness. If you experience these reactions, discontinue use and contact your health practitioner.

ELDERBERRY
(*Sambucus nigra*)

Overall Rating . . . . *Highly Recommended*

For healing burns, including sunburn . . *Highly Recommended*

For treating cuts and wounds . . . . *Highly Recommended*

For conditioning the skin . . . . *Recommended*

To alleviate the symptoms of
digestive disorders . . . . *Recommended*

Here's a clue that might stump even the most dedicated *Jeopardy* fan: "Different parts of this plant can be used to call elk, dye hair black, build a popgun, make chutney, and fight the flu." Got any ideas? How about, "What is elderberry?"

To elaborate, elderberry is a bushy plant that has traditionally been used for a wide range of household and medicinal purposes. Commonly used to fight the flu, hayfever, colds, and coughs, a compound found in elderberry flowers and berries prevents viruses from invading the respiratory system. An article in *Pediatric News* in 1997 praised elderberry for its flu-fighting abilities.

So, if you're feeling slightly ill or if you have a full-blown cold, drink three cups of elderberry tea per day for a couple of days. The tea, especially good if mixed with yarrow or peppermint, should have you feeling better. Or take two 500-milligram capsules per day for up to four days.

Elderberry jelly or a few spoonfuls of elderberry juice can help you through a bout of constipation and is safe for children. If you have minor cuts or burns, a compress of elderberry juice and honey (to act as a thickener) may offer some relief. You get a superficial cut out in the woods? Try putting some flowers directly on your wound to help stop the bleeding and ease the pain. If you suffer from hemorrhoids or just want an excuse for a leisurely, relaxing soak, try mixing elderberry tea (alone or in combination with honeysuckle tea) or elderberry flowers into your next bath. Victorian women swore by the relaxing powers of elderberry—flower water was a staple of the dressing table.

 ## RECOMMENDED USAGE

There is no RDI for elderberry.

Children
Administer only under the advice of a doctor or health practitioner.

Adults
Capsules
Two 375-milligram capsules up to three times daily.
Tea
One cup no more than three times daily.
Tincture
Three drops in an 8-ounce glass of water three times daily.

 ## CAUTION!

Don't eat elderberry roots, stems, or leaves, as they are poisonous. Raw berries may make you sick, but once they are cooked, they are harmless.

ELECTROLYTES
(Potassium, Sodium, and Chloride)

Overall Recommendation . . . . *Highly Recommended*

To rehydrate the body . . . . *Highly Recommended*

Dancing the tango is a fine art. As the sultry music begins to rise, the dancers engage in a breathtaking balancing act—each responsible for their own moves while somehow gliding across the floor as a single organism. So imagine the electrolytes potassium, sodium, and chloride involved in some complicated choreography of their own. In a promenade that never stops, they dance around and with one another in order to keep the cells of our body in balance.

Electrolytes are water-soluble minerals that charge our cells with electricity. Potassium and sodium have positive charges, while chloride has a negative charge. These electric properties give electrolytes free passage in and out of our cells to deliver glucose—the food cells thrive on—and take out extra water and waste. Our cells require a balance between the potassium within their walls and the sodium swishing around in the fluids just outside. If too much of either electrolyte builds up, they both shift back and forth until balance is regained. Chloride, meanwhile, bonds with sodium to concoct a formula similar to table salt, which in turn makes hydrochloric acid, the substance that digests food in our stomach. Working as a team, our electrolytes are necessary for

* keeping blood pressure levels and heartbeat steady
* delivering impulse messages to the nerves

✸ balancing the body's water levels

✸ equalizing the internal balance of acid and alkaline

✸ releasing hormones

Electrolytes are most commonly lost when the body is at a period of internal imbalance, such as diarrhea. In this case, both the American Medical Association and the American Pediatric Association recommend replacing lost fluids with electolytes. Often, the easiest way to do this is with an electrolyte beverage such as Gatorade or Pedialyte.

Most of us know that too much sodium can increase blood pressure. Potassium helps counteract this effect. But keep in mind that too much sodium can inhibit potassium levels. Using potassium to lower blood pressure therefore works best when sodium is simultaneously reduced. A benefit of keeping blood pressure at a healthy rate is that it lessens the risk of heart disease and kidney trouble. Because potassium does such a good job of regulating the heart, it may also protect us from strokes.

The electrolytes sodium and chloride are prevalent in most foods. In fact, don't go out of your way to eat them, because most of us normally get too much of these substances in our diets anyway.

On the other hand, it's easy to lose potassium from our bodies, though vital to keep it well-stocked so the all-important dance of the electrolytes can keep us in good shape. The finest sources of potassium are beans, veggies, and fruits. Some potassium-packed choices include avocados, bananas, black beans, cantaloupes, garbanzo beans, kidney beans, lentils, mint leaves, orange juice, baked potatoes (skin included), prune juice, raisins, sunflower seeds, sweet potatoes, tomato juice, and watercress.

RECOMMENDED USAGE

There is no RDI for electrolytes.

Children
Administer only under the advice of a doctor or health practitioner.

Adults
RDIs have not been established for electrolytes, and the only one of the three that needs to be supplemented is potassium. Foods, however, remain the best source for potassium. That's because regulations governing supplements limit the amount of potassium available in each pill or capsule. As a result, buying supplements could be expensive, not to mention cause stomach upset and supply us with no more potassium than we might get from a few bites of a baked potato or a handful of sunflower seeds.

And remember—increasing potassium only helps if you keep it in balance with sodium. Nutritionists suggest a 1 to 1 ratio of potassium and sodium for optimum health.

 CAUTION!

If you consume lots of coffee, alcohol, and sugar, or are stressed out and at the same time feel run down and weak in the knees and have muscle cramps, your potassium levels may be low. Being sick, on an extremely low carbohydrate diet, or anorexic, may cause nausea and rapid heartbeat. In extreme cases, electrolyte depletion can even lead to heart failure. Because vomiting and diarrhea deplete electrolytes, children with these symptoms must be kept hydrated.

Medications that heavily interfere with potassium are diuretics and prescription drugs used to treat heart problems. Balancing potassium and heart medication isn't easy and could have lethal effects. Consult with your health care practitioner before mixing these two substances.

Exceeding 18 grams of potassium is toxic and fatal. You'd have to work hard to ingest this much, though, and it wouldn't be from your food. This kind of overdose mostly happens with people who have kidney problems or who improperly use supplements.

EUCALYPTUS
(*Eucalyptus globulus*)

Overall Rating . . . . *Highly Recommended*

For treating respiratory conditions . . . *Highly Recommended*

Unknown in Europe and North American until the colonization of Australia in the nineteenth century, the stately, blue-gray eucalyptus tree was a staple of aboriginal life for centuries. Used medicinally for everything from breaking a fever to cleansing a wound, the extensive hollow root systems of this tree were also relied on by the aborigines for water, while the twigs and peeling bark were used for cleansing their bodies and teeth. The leaves are edible, too, although they tend to be preferred by koalas, who spend much of their lives in these trees, munching.

You've most likely experienced the expectorant power of eucalyptus when you've had a cold or cough. A popular ingredient in throat lozenges and chest rubs, eucalyptus puts the *lyptus* in "mentho-lyptus" drops and adds the heat and vapors to the rub in small jars of "vapo-rubs." And not only is eucalyptus effective at breaking up mucus, but when the crushed leaves or oil are inhaled, their antiseptic properties may also help fight colds, sinus infections, pneumonia, and other upper respiratory problems. If you've got a cold and are not inclined to purchase one of the many over-the-counter products containing eucalyptus, you might want to try a weak tea made from eucalyptus leaves.

When used in massage oils, eucalyptus may help soothe arthritis, while a bath enhanced by eucalyptus leaves may help alleviate everyday aches and pains. In addition to being a natural antiseptic, eucalyptus is antifungal, which may make it effective against conditions like athlete's foot and lice. It is also useful for cleaning sores, minor wounds, and insect bites.

 ## RECOMMENDED USAGE

There is no RDI for eucalyptus.

To treat respiratory discomforts associated with colds, flu, asthma, or allergies, combine 1 to 2 milliliters of eucalyptus oil in 25 milliliters of carrier oil. Rub on chest. Combine with essential oils of thyme, lemon balm, fennel, peppermint, or anise to elevate antiseptic and expectorant properties. Add ten drops of oil in steaming water for an effective inhalant.

 ## CAUTION!

Eucalyptus oil is toxic and is for external use only. Even when applied topically, undiluted eucalyptus oil can cause nausea, diarrhea, vomiting, skin irritation, and muscle spasms. Use extra caution and get a doctor's approval before administering to children. A good rule of thumb: The oil should always be diluted with no more than 2 teaspoons per pint of water, vegetable oil, or rubbing alcohol. Keep eucalyptus oil away from your eyes and use only a half dose when pregnant. Eucalyptus tea should also be well diluted before you drink it.

EVENING PRIMROSE OIL

Overall Rating . . . . *Highly Recommended*

For relieving symptoms of PMS . . . . . *Highly Recommended*

For treating eczema . . . . *Recommended*

To lower cholesterol and
blood pressure . . . . *Highly Recommended*

To prevent cancer . . . . *Recommended*

If you're a woman, you might be familiar with these symptoms: You feel a little bloated. You're grouchy. Or weepy. You can't cope with even a small glass of spilled milk. Or maybe it's just about craving chocolate—but craving it like you'd do anything for it.

No, it's not in your head. Premenstrual syndrome (PMS) is very real and upsets the lives of millions of women (and their loved ones) every month. For many of these women, evening primrose oil is often a saving grace when nothing else seems to work.

An all-American hailing from Virginia, this beneficial oil is pressed from the seeds of the yellow-flowered evening primrose plant. The main reason this oil has such therapeutic effects is because it's high in gamma linolenic acid, an omega-6 essential fatty acid known—among other things—for reducing inflammation in the uterus. Hence, relief from PMS.

When this herb was introduced to Europe in the seventeenth century, it was hailed as a cure-all. And though it's not quite that, people keep reaching for evening primrose oil not only because it may relieve the symptoms of PMS, but because it also might

- soothe the itching, oozing, and redness of eczema—even allowing some people to reduce the use of steroid medications
- help lower cholesterol and blood pressure
- keep hair, skin, and fingernails supple and strong

Evening primrose oil may be effective in treating mild cases of rheumatoid arthritis and is also thought to slow the progress of multiple sclerosis.

When babies get cradle cap (a form of eczema that turns their scalps itchy, red, and scaly), evening primrose oil is a natural way to bring relief. But don't give it to them orally; only use it topically.

Had a little too much fun last night? Evening primrose oil helps with hangovers. Tired of having too much to drink too often? Evening primrose oil may also help you kick alcohol altogether, since it cleans up the liver more quickly. Alcoholics report that it helps them quit cold turkey because it makes their minds sharper.

Most interestingly, though, is a study from the mid 1980s that indicates evening primrose oil (as well as other EFAs) is effective in reversing the cancer-causing effects of radiation and carcinogens.

It can be purchased in both oil and capsule form and is widely available in most health food stores. For topical use, simply open one of the capsules and apply it where needed.

 RECOMMENDED USAGE

There is no RDI for evening primrose oil.

Children
Administer only under the advice of a doctor or health practitioner.

Adults

Capsules

One 250-milligram capsule up to three times daily.

Liquid

One to three drops in an 8-ounce glass of water, up to three times daily.

Women

For premenstrual symptoms, two 500-milligram capsules two to three times daily.

 CAUTION!

Evening primrose oil is nontoxic, but it may have a few adverse effects. Even though this oil is a good source of GLA, the most beneficial omega-6 essential fatty acid, it also contains a lot of linoleic acid, which can cause inflammation. So if you suffer from arthritis, asthma, or migraines, taking evening primrose oil could make your symptoms worse. The same is true of people who have epilepsy. For them, seizures could result. If any of these descriptions apply to you, evening primrose oil is probably not the best choice.

Taken on an empty stomach, evening primrose oil can cause nausea. When first introduced, it might cause upset stomach, headaches, and acne. Sometimes taking the supplement with food and giving your body time to adjust can ease these symptoms. But if these suggestions don't help, discontinue use.

FENNEL
(*Foeniculum vulgare*)

Overall Rating . . . . *Recommended*

For treating gastrointestinal disorders . . . . . . *Recommended*

Throw some in a green salad to add an unusual flair. Spice up fish dishes with it to delight your palate. Chew on it after an Indian meal to calm the spices once they reach your stomach. These are the most common ways we utilize the good flavor and settling effects of fennel. There's a lot more to the fennel story, however.

Fennel is now grown in the United States, the Mediterranean region, and Asia, but back when it was known almost solely to the Greeks, it was given to people considered overweight, as it was thought to be an appetite suppressant. The British used to hand out fennel during church services, especially during times of fasting, to quiet the rumblings of congregation tummies.

Although the berries, root, fruit, and stem of the fennel plant can be utilized, the seeds are most effective for its medicinal purposes. Either chewing on the seeds or drinking a decoction or tea from them can help treat

- bad breath
- indigestion or gas
- irritable bowel syndrome
- low milk production in lactating mothers
- PMS breast pain

❦ high anxiety

❦ coughs or colds

Pouring the essential oil into water to produce a vaporizer can also assist in treating other respiratory problems, as well as help detoxify the body. In fact, bathing in water to which fennel oil has been added is considered an excellent way to cleanse the body of toxins.

 RECOMMENDED USAGE

There is no RDI for fennel.

Children
Not advised for children. Administer only under the advice of a doctor or health practitioner.

Adults
Capsules
One 100-milligram capsule up to three times daily.
Tincture
Three drops in an 8-ounce glass of water three times daily.

Fennel seeds can be found at most health food stores and when in season in grocery stores.

To increase breast milk production, simply chew on the seeds or make some tea. To make fennel tea, pour 2 cups of boiling water over 1 teaspoon of fennel seeds.

To relieve tired eyes, take 1 teaspoon of fennel powder (ground-up seeds) to 2 ounces of cold water. Strain water and use for eyewash. This may also help conjunctivitis.

To eliminate gas or indigestion, drink 1 cup of tea before meals.

Add fennel oil to the bath to relieve muscular aches and pains or symptoms of rheumatism.

 CAUTION!

Fennel is a uterine stimulant. Don't use it during pregnancy. If you have chronic trouble with your gastrointestinal tract, avoid fennel.

If you have very sensitive skin or are prone to allergies, avoid using the oil.

FENUGREEK

Overall Rating . . . . *Recommended*

To increase sexual energy . . . . *Not Recommended*
For calming upset stomach . . . . *Recommended*

On a list that includes oysters, grapes, gingko nuts, vanilla, and romantic, candlelit dinners, some might add the herb fenugreek. Fenugreek is one of those ancient herbs that's tried and true—Hippocrates was a fan—and has quite an array of uses. Its medicinal purposes include

- regulating blood sugar
- lowering cholesterol
- reducing abdominal cramps associated with menstruation and diarrhea
- settling upset stomachs
- treating menstrual and menopausal problems related to kidney weakness.

In addition, fenugreek can be used to increase the flow of breast milk, clear mucous congestion, ease coughing and sore throats, soothe irritated and inflamed skin, and act as a bulking laxative. It has been used for thousands of years to combat indigestion and upset stomachs.

Because it's one of the most ancient medicinal herbs, fenugreek is well known in China, Egypt, the Middle East, and the Balkans. Although its numerous uses may not provide relief in all cases, it doesn't hurt to give fenugreek a try since it's virtually harmless.

If you're struggling with menstrual cramps or stomach upsets, boil some fenugreek seeds in water for an hour; then strain and drink the decoction. This helps increase the flow of milk during breastfeeding, says Jay N. Gordon, M.D., F.A.A.P., a pediatric and nutrition specialist in Santa Monica, California. In addition, for easing abdominal cramps and menstrual pain, try making a tea out of the leaves and stems. If you've got blood sugar troubles, drink tincture or swallow a capsules of fenugreek. Is your skin inflamed? Take loose powder or powder from capsules and mix with water to turn into a paste. Apply directly on the inflammation.

This herb is available in tinctures, capsules, and crushed seeds (good for gargling when you have a sore throat).

 RECOMMENDED USAGE

There is no RDI for fenugreek.

Children
Administer only under the advice of a doctor or health practitioner.

Adults
Capsules
One to three capsules three times daily.
Tincture
Two to four drops in water up to three times daily.
Gargle
Mix 1 tablespoon of crushed seeds in 8 ounces of hot water. Use every three to four hours for relief.

CAUTION!

If you're pregnant or trying to conceive, don't use fenugreek. It stimulates the uterus and could cause problems. Fenugreek is also thought to help regulate blood sugar, but diabetics who use insulin should first consult with a professional before using fenugreek for this purpose.

Fenugreek is nontoxic.

FEVERFEW

Overall Rating . . . . *Recommended*

**For treating migraines and
other headaches** . . . . *Recommended*

For alleviating arthritis pain . . . . *Not Recommended*

Although they may seem like a thoroughly modern response to the pressures of our time, headaches have always plagued humankind. But what did we do before pain and headache medications were so readily available? As far back as ancient Greece, we employed the feverfew plant, with its feathery white petals surrounding a sunny yellow orb. Most widely celebrated for its ability to treat migraine headaches, feverfew is also beneficial for the female reproductive system and may help alleviate the symptoms of rheumatoid arthritis.

Migraine headaches are doozies. Referred to as vascular headaches because they involve the blood vessels in the head, migraines can be debilitating until they pass hours or even days later. But studies at the London Migraine Clinic and one reported in the *Lancet* have good news for migraine sufferers. These studies have determined that feverfew blocks serotonin, which is emitted from blood platelets, as well as prostaglandins released by red blood cells. Both of these hormonelike substances have an inflammatory effect and result in head pain, sensitivity to light, a prickly feeling in the limbs, visual disturbances, nausea, and vomiting—in short, a migraine.

It takes some time—usually about three months—but taking

feverfew on a regular basis can help relieve and even prevent these symptoms. About 80 percent of the people who use it report an improvement in their symptoms, but clinical data have yet to back this up.

Because feverfew treats inflammation, it's been used to tone the uterus after childbirth, stimulate uterine contractions, and relieve menstrual pain. The herb may also help relieve the pain and swelling of rheumatoid arthritis, due to its ability to inhibit pro-inflammatory prostaglandins.

Other speculated uses for feverfew include reducing fever, treating insect bites, and getting rid of worms.

This herb may be found dried as well as in tincture and capsule forms.

 ## RECOMMENDED USAGE

There is no RDI for feverfew.

Children
Administer only under the advice of a doctor or health practitioner.

Adults
Capsules
One to three 380-milligram capsules up to three times daily.

 ## CAUTION!

People who eat fresh leaves off the feverfew plant may experience mouth ulcers. Try sautéing the leaves to prevent the problem. If that doesn't help, stop eating them and consult a health care practitioner.

Feverfew is a natural blood thinner, so it's not recommended for people taking blood-thinning medications, as it could lead to dangerously thin blood.

Injecting feverfew, which is uncommon, has been known to cause a life-threatening allergic reaction called anaphylaxis. Anaphylaxis is characterized by extreme itching, pallor, and a drop in blood pressure, followed by unconsciousness and maybe even a coma. Even though it's not common, a reaction such as this requires immediate assistance—call 911 right away.

FLAXSEED OIL

Overall Rating.................. *Highly Recommended*

To stunt the growth of
cancerous tumors............... *Recommended*

For reducing heart problems........ *Highly Recommended*

To relieve inflammation .... *Recommended*

For alleviating symptoms of
menopause.................... *Highly Recommended*

If you don't mind the wrinkles, there's nothing more stylish on a
hot day than a fine linen garment—especially, it seems, when on
safari. At least that's what the travel brochures would have you
think. But aside from keeping hot-climate dwellers cool, flax—the
source of linen fiber—is also in demand for its oil. Flaxseed oil,
also called linseed oil, has a number of medicinal uses because it

* is a major source of the essential fatty acids cis-linoleic and
  alpha-linolenic
* potentially stunts the growth of tumors, particularly in breast,
  colon, and lung cancer
* helps relieve inflammation caused by allergies, arthritis, psoriasis, and the like
* cools hot flashes during menopause and normalizes hormone
  levels
* fights bacteria, fungi, and viruses

Flaxseed oil is one of the most commonly prescribed supplements today, according to Dean Ornish, M.D., author of *Reversing*

Heart Disease. This is because flaxseed oil corrects fatty acid imbalances that may cause heart problems and is also an easy substance to ingest.

Part of what makes flaxseed oil so beneficial is that it's our largest source of lignans. Lignans are plant fibers that get transformed during digestion into unique cancer-fighting and hormone-regulating compounds. It's also speculated that flaxseed oil can help silken dry skin, while the whole seeds may be useful as a bulking laxative or as an elixir for sore throats. Flax seeds are also popular in poultices, which are applied on the chest to relieve the symptoms of a cold.

 ## RECOMMENDED USAGE

There is no RDI for flaxseed oil.

Children
Administer only under the advice of a doctor or health practitioner.

Adults
Flaxseed oil supplements are widely available in the form of capsules and oils, and some nutritionists suggest taking up to three 1,000-milligram capsules, or 2 tablespoonfuls of the oil, each day.

 ## CAUTION!

One of the biggest concerns about flaxseed oil is rancidity. This substance is very hard to maintain and has a reputation for turning rancid quite quickly. Preparation is also important and could mean the difference between getting something that will boost your health or potentially cause you harm.

When buying a flaxseed supplement, certain information on the label can be used as a guideline for knowing whether or not you have a good product. The best oils will have the endorsement of a third party, which certifies it is organic. It's best to stay away from "cold pressed" oils because, like partially hydrogenated oil, the process involved artificially changes the structure of the essential fatty acids. The safest extraction methods are by expeller pressing or by a process called modified atmospheric packing. Again, this should be listed on the label.

Both light and heat spoil flaxseed oil, so seek out products in dark-colored bottles, which keep the light out, and if your health food store keeps flaxseed products refrigerated, all the better. Finally, taste is one of the best indicators. If you're left with a bitter aftertaste or it just tastes spoiled, then it is. If there's no taste at all, it's probably too refined to do much good.

Flaxseed oil, if taken in large amounts, can have potentially toxic effects. That's because the seeds carry a slight trace of prussic acid, though no cases of prussic acid poisoning have been recorded. Artists use a form of linseed oil in their paints, and this is definitely not to be ingested. Flaxseed toxicity can result in convulsions, shortness of breath, excitability, and weakness. If you encounter any of these symptoms, stop taking the supplement immediately and seek professional medical assistance.

Flaxseed oil may also inhibit the body's ability to absorb iron and other minerals, though this is not considered a major concern.

Finally, pregnant and breastfeeding women are advised not to use flaxseed oil, as the potential dangers are not worth the risk of endangering a pregnancy.

FOLATE
(Folic Acid)

Overall Rating . . . . *Highly Recommended*

For fetal development . . . . *Highly Recommended*

To prevent heart attacks . . . . *Highly Recommended*

For treating osteoporosis . . . . *Highly Recommended*

Ask any parent-to-be their most heartfelt wish, and they'll respond without hesitation: a healthy baby. The happy answer to their prayer is due, in part, to folate—also called folic acid. Another of the B vitamins, this substance is vital to the development and upkeep of each and every one of our cells.

Folate is essential for producing RNA and DNA, the genetic "specs" that help determine how each of us turns out. On a broader scale, folate helps red blood cells form as they should, while also ensuring that body cells divide and replicate. Since the human fetus is a sophisticated exercise in cell division, replication, and growth, you can see just how important folate is.

Folic acid also plays a significant role in a number of other body processes such as

- working with vitamin B_{12} to metabolize sugar and amino acids
- synthesizing proteins, also in conjunction with vitamin B_{12}
- proper functioning of neurotransmitters
- mobilizing and strengthening white blood cells and antibodies
- preventing arteries from clogging

🕸 regulating embryonic and fetal nerve cell formation
🕸 ensuring healthy development of sex organs

Folate is most often used to promote healthy function of the female reproductive system. Dysplasia, a condition in which borderline abnormal tissue grows around the cervix, can increase a woman's risk for cervical cancer. Folate often helps prevent such growth from recurring. On the other end of the spectrum, pregnancy asks a lot of a woman's body and sometimes results in anemia. Here, too, folate can give those red blood cells a much needed lift. Folate used alongside vitamin B_{12} is also widely known to prevent birth defects, particularly those affecting the brain, spinal cord, and nervous system, and is officially recommended by the American Medical Association for all women of childbearing age.

Researchers have discovered that elevated homocysteine levels are a major risk factor for both heart attacks and osteoporosis. Folic acid has been found to reduce homocysteine, particularly when combined with vitamins B_{12} and B_6.

On top of these many significant functions, folic acid is speculated to relieve minor body aches and pains, ward off depression, improve lactation, brighten skin tone, and prevent canker sores.

Folate is naturally found in lots of great-tasting foods. Dark green leafy veggies, including spinach, kale, endive, and collard greens, top the list. Different kinds of beans, such as garbanzo, soy, peas, and lentils, are high in folic acid, and other plant sources include apricots, asparagus, avocados, barley, brewer's yeast, broccoli, cantaloupes, carrots, pumpkins, rice, sprouts, and wheat germ. Liver—be it beef, chicken, lamb, or pork—and eggs also have folic acid. It's important to know, however, that only about a quarter of the folic acid in our food is available to us. This is due to folate's chemical makeup, and then aggravated by the way we cook and process foods.

RECOMMENDED USAGE

Children
50–150 micrograms

Adults
180–200 micrograms

All women of child bearing age: 400–800 micrograms

Due to information that continues to surface about the positive effects of folate, most nutritionists think the current RDIs are too low and expect they will soon go up. In fact, many experts suggest a daily minimum of 400 micrograms of folate for adults and 800 micrograms for pregnant and lactating women.

 CAUTION!

As critical as folate is to so many processes, it's also sensitive to a number of factors. People most susceptible to folic acid deficiency include women who are pregnant, breastfeeding, or use oral contraceptives, and anyone who abuses alcohol, smokes cigarettes, has a diet lacking in calories and nutrients or can't digest properly, and those recovering from an operation or major illness. These conditions stress the body and deplete folate reserves.

Medications can also reduce folate levels by preventing absorption. The most common folate inhibitors include aspirin, seizure medications, antibiotics, and anesthetics.

A folate deficiency will most likely reveal itself through a unique form of anemia that causes short-lived, oversized, and uneven red blood cells. Other symptoms may include feeling weak, irritable, listless, and nauseous, as well as being unable to sleep.

In the case of anemia, it's crucial to have a blood test to determine whether the cause is a folate deficiency or a B_{12} deficiency. The reason for this is that folate supplements will make B_{12} anemia appear to vanish, when in fact it has not. Neurological damage could then result.

Folate is nontoxic unless taken in high doses of more than 1,500 micrograms per day. Over time, folate at such extremes could cause harmful folacin crystals to build up in the kidneys. Other complaints may include stomach upset, gas, and bloating. Anyone considering such high doses of folic acid should consult a health practitioner.

PREGNANCY

Vitamin and mineral supplementation during pregnancy is essential to the mother's health, as well as to the health of her growing baby. A prenatal vitamin that contains the needed nutritional supplementation during pregnancy is an important addition to a pregnant woman's diet. Studies show that, by taking supplements, the incidence of a low-birth-weight baby decreases, the risk of a neural tube defect such as spina bifida is dramatically reduced, mental and physical retardation are reduced; the baby's skeletal development is improved, and pregnancy complications are reduced.

The best approach is to take a multiple vitamin and mineral supplement. An ideal prenatal supplement would include

❧ Vitamin A—800 RE (retinol equivalents, equal to 1 microgram of retinol or 6 micrograms of beta-carotene)

- Beta-carotene—10 milligrams
- Vitamin D—10 micrograms
- Vitamin E—20 milligrams
- Vitamin B_1—1.5 milligrams
- Vitamin B_2—1.6 milligrams
- Niacin—17 milligrams
- Vitamin B_6—2.2 milligrams
- Folic acid—400 micrograms
- Vitamin B_{12}—2.2 micrograms
- Vitamin C—70 milligrams
- Calcium—1,000 milligrams
- Chromium—100 micrograms
- Copper—1.5milligrams
- Fluoride—2.0 milligrams
- Iodine—175 micrograms
- Iron—30–60 milligrams
- Magnesium—320 milligrams
- Molybdenum—100 micrograms
- Selenium—65 micrograms
- Zinc—15 milligrams[1]

Additionally, your doctor may recommend a greater intake of iron, calcium, or magnesium, depending on your diet and your health.

[1] Somer, E. *Nutrition for a Healthy Pregnancy,* Owl Books, 1995.

GARLIC
(*Allium sativum*)

Overall Rating. . . . . *Highly Recommended*

To reduce cholesterol . . . . *Not Recommended*

To lower blood pressure. . . . . *Recommended*

For the immune system . . . . *Highly Recommended*

This tiny, potent bulb has been treasured since antiquity for its culinary and therapeutic uses. The ancient Greeks and Romans used garlic medicinally but also believed it protected them in times of war and strife. Egyptian slaves working on the pyramids ate garlic to increase their stamina. The Chinese valued garlic for its ability to improve circulation and strengthen the heart. In the Middle Ages, people believed garlic protected against the plague, and in central Europe it was used to repel vampires.

In the twentieth century, on the battlefields of both world wars, garlic was applied to wounds to ward off infection. Today, many of the claims regarding garlic's medicinal powers seem to be borne out. Generally safe, with few, if any, side effects beyond bad breath (and many people don't even mind its smell), who would imagine that this unassuming clove could pack such a powerful pharmaceutical punch?

A relative of the onion, garlic is a natural antibiotic. When garlic is crushed, the antibiotic allicin is formed. Allicin is equal in strength to 1 percent penicillin, and while it probably won't work as quickly as penicillin, it does appear to have broad-spectrum effectiveness in fighting infections. Garlic is also an effective antiseptic, antifungal, and antimicrobial treatment. Garlic juice or crushed garlic placed on a wound or infected insect bite could

- promote healing
- reduce pain and irritation
- soothe burns
- treat acne

Garlic juice or capsules can also combat fungal infections like athlete's foot and thrush. In addition, garlic works on viruses that manifest as herpes simplex and influenza.

Many experts believe garlic plays a vital role in maintaining a proper bacterial balance in the intestines. Drinking garlic juice straight or steeped in milk may be helpful in ridding the intestines of yeasts or parasites, both in humans and animals. Eating crushed garlic or taking garlic capsules may also ease gastroenteritis and traveler's diarrhea.

Garlic has long been effective as an expectorant to help treat coughs and bronchitis. Crushed garlic steeped in honey makes an almost tasty cough syrup that children can take. Blend olive oil and garlic for a chest rub to ease lung problems or for ear drops to fight off an earache (except if there's any chance the eardrum may be perforated). And, if you can brave walking around with major garlic breath, go ahead and eat several cloves a day—it's a real boon to the immune system, as proven by a 1983 study researching the health benefits of garlic and onions.

Chomping down a clove a day could also kill off a cold, reduce a fever, or simply battle against allergies or unwanted germs that may be wandering around your house or office. Part of why garlic is so good for us is that it contains antioxidants that may provide protection against stomach and other cancers. It's potentially helpful in regulating blood sugar levels, thus easing or helping to prevent late-onset diabetes. And if you're concerned about your heart and circulatory system, garlic may help reduce blood pressure, although speculation that it reduces serum cholesterol levels was recently dashed in mid-1998 by a German study reported in the *Journal of the American Medical Association*. Garlic has also been shown to reduce the risk of blood clots, dangerous deposits from the blood vessels, and the risk of a second heart attack.

And finally–wouldn't you know it?–potent and odiferous, garlic can also be used in place of smelling salts!

Incorporating garlic into your daily diet is an easy—and delicious—way to increase your intake. Crush it over salads, cook it with meats, add it to sauces and soups, and distill it into syrups, oils, and tinctures.

Most of us prefer chewing gum rather than garlic, but beware that cooking it, and especially boiling it, does reduce its potency. But if you do eat it raw and notice that whenever you speak to someone, their eyes start to water and they plug their nose, eat some parsley or even a strawberry to offset the odor. You can try garlic capsules instead of eating it fresh, but some deodorized garlic products are useless, because the therapeutic power of garlic comes from the smelly sulfur-containing compounds. Some believe that without that distinctive smell, it'll lose its effectiveness.

 ## RECOMMENDED USAGE

There is no RDI for garlic.

Children
Administer only under the advice of a doctor or health practitioner.

Adults
Capsules
One 400-milligram capsule up to three times daily with meals.

Cloves
Two to three cloves daily.

To reduce cholesterol, take a supplement equivalent to 4,000 milligrams of fresh garlic daily.

 CAUTION!

Although generally safe, garlic isn't recommended for children under three years of age. In addition, it can cause heartburn or an upset stomach, especially in pregnant women. Nursing mothers are generally advised not to take therapeutic doses of garlic, as this may upset their babies. Some pediatricians, however, believe that taking garlic actually entices a baby to drink more milk. In fact, a 1995 study found that infants offered garlic-flavored breast milk actually nursed longer. Taking garlic, how much, and in what form, is definitely a matter of personal taste.

GERANIUM
(*Pelargonium odorantissimum*)

Overall Rating . . . . *Recommended*

For relaxation and revitalization
(aromatherapy) . . . . *Recommended*

To treat digestive problems. . . . . *Recommended*

To apply as a topical analgesic . . . . *Recommended*

Nothing announces the arrival of summer as surely as the appearance of a terra-cotta pot full of jolly red geraniums. While you're probably familiar with the plant on a sun deck, porch, or patio, the geranium is also found in a different form in the wild, with two flowers on a long fragile stem. This wild geranium is actually a species of flower known as cranesbill, or American cranesbill (*Geranium maculatum*), and has different herbal and medicinal uses than those of what is popularly called the geranium. Using the names *geranium* and *cranesbill* to avoid confusion, we'll cover the uses of both plants.

Geranium is generally used in oil form for massage and aromatherapy. Geranium oil has soothing and revitalizing properties. It can be rubbed onto tired limbs or the back for a recharge. Rubbed onto the breasts, geranium oil can help ease the pain of mastitis, according to French studies. When poured into a bath, geranium oil is thought to act as an analgesic, easing the discomfort associated with conditions such as shingles and eczema. This oil can also be applied sparingly to burns.

Geranium oil is frequently used in perfumes and combines well with many citrus and floral essential oils. Feeling stressed? Place a tiny amount of geranium oil in a vaporizer or small bowl and let its scent relax and revive your frazzled nerves. You might also want to try putting several drops of oil in hand lotion and using it as a pick-me-up when you're feeling blue. Finally, if you are heading off into the woods for several days of backpacking or camping, geranium oil would be a handy (and lightweight) addition to your pack to use both as a deodorant and an insect repellent.

Cranesbill is one of many astringent herbs that some believe is useful for toning and firming tissue, reducing discharges (mucus, for example), and arresting bleeding. Cranesbill is generally not taken alone but in combination with other herbs that have complementary properties.

The leaves and roots of cranesbill are most commonly used as ingredients in teas designed to ease the symptoms of diarrhea. Look for cranesbill in combination with herbs such as bayberry, oak bark, and meadowsweet. Cranesbill is thought to act by strengthening intestinal tissue and may also be helpful to people suffering from duodenal ulcers and colitis. Cranesbill, again in combination with other herbs, can be used to help relieve excessive bleeding during menstruation. However, herbal teas are not meant to cure any of these conditions, each of which can be serious. If your symptoms persist, it is best to consult your health care provider.

 ## RECOMMENDED USAGE

There is no RDI for geranium.

Children
Administer only under the advice of a doctor or health practitioner.

Adults

Essential oil

As desired, in bath or infuser.

Capsules

One 100-milligram capsule up to three times daily.

Topically

Apply as needed.

 CAUTION!

Geranium and cranesbill have very different uses and should not be confused. Geranium essential oil is not generally recommended for internal use, while cranesbill is an ingredient found in many medicinal teas and tinctures. Products containing cranesbill are generally safe for children and the elderly. Excessive use of cranesbill, however, can cause constipation and stiff joints. In addition, if symptoms of diarrhea, digestive upset, intestinal bleeding, or heavy menstrual periods persist for more than several days, check with your doctor.

Infants, children, and pregnant women should use geranium oil sparingly, after diluting it to half strength. It should not be used at all by people with tumors.

GINGER
(*Zingiber officinale*)

Overall Rating . . . . *Recommended*

For reducing morning sickness . . . . *Recommended*

For preventing motion sickness. . . . . *Recommended*

For easing nausea. *Recommended*

Bake it into sweets! Turn it into candy! Distill it into hot and cold drinks! Season the most savory of foods with it! No wonder people name their babies after this versatile, delicious herb. And, no wonder it's such a common ingredient in Chinese, Eastern, Caribbean, and African cuisine.

Deemed helpful for ailments ranging from chilblains (skin irritation and burning resulting from exposure to moist cold) to morning sickness, ginger is also one of the most typically used herbs in Chinese medicine. One reason is that there are so many ways to take it: in teas, tinctures, powders and oils—even added to food, it can deliver a good therapeutic punch. On top of all that, it's easy to find and generally one of the least expensive items in the produce section of most grocery stores.

Preventing and easing nausea is one of the most popular uses of this wonderful herb. Whether you want to prevent motion sickness, reduce morning sickness, or settle an upset stomach, ginger capsules and ginger tea are widely used antinauseants. (While you shouldn't binge on ginger during pregnancy, it's still considered safe for the fetus in small doses.) In fact, ginger is widely becoming the most prescribed antinausea "drug" today. An article in the medical journal *Current Opinion in Obstetrics and Gynecology* recommended ginger as a safe and effective treatment for nausea and vomiting during pregnancy.

It's also safe for kids and easy to get them to take. Before your next car trip, bake a batch of ginger cookies and let your little darlings munch their way to your destination. If that sounds like too much work, chewing on a piece of crystallized ginger (widely available as a baking spice) or drinking ginger ale made from real ginger can also do the trick.

For people undergoing surgery or chemotherapy, ginger doesn't seem to interfere with medication and can help offset the nausea resulting from anesthesia or the chemotherapy.

Even with all its obvious straightforward uses, ginger is a bit of a paradox. For example, even though it's pungent to the nose and taste buds, it calms and soothes digestive upsets like gas and heartburn.

It is also thought to work as an effective pain reliever, easing muscular aches and pains, stiff joints, arthritis, cramps, toothache, and headache. Try this the next time you come home stiff and sore from overexertion or illness: Boil some grated ginger and soak a towel in the warm liquid. Place the towel on the painful area, lie down, and relax. Ginger is thought to increase the flow of blood to where it's applied, and this may dull the pain and ease out any tension. Drinking a bit of hot ginger tea at the same time may promote healing both inside and out.

If you've got a cold, hot ginger tea may help stimulate your immune system, while at the same time reduce fever, cough, and pain. Try some peppermint tea with ginger and clove added to it or chamomile tea with ginger, honey, and lemon. This tea is especially useful for coughs and laryngitis, and once it has cooled a bit, try gargling with it to ease a sore throat. Even if you're not sick, on a cold wintry day a cup of ginger tea may warm your body by increasing circulation and promoting perspiration.

Because of ginger's strong warming properties, a footbath infused with it may both warm you and ease the pain of chilblains. Ginger powder sprinkled into your shoes may prevent chilblains and keep your feet warm. Other uses of ginger include easing the symptoms of asthma, combating yeast infections, and boosting male fertility.

According to Earl Mindell, M.D., author of *The Herb Bible,* experts agree that ginger can also help prevent atherosclerosis, or hardening of the arteries, by reducing cholesterol levels and slowing the development of plaque in the arteries. Adding ginger to the food you eat, especially to meat, is an easy way to realize the benefits—and culinary delights—of this incredible root.

 ## RECOMMENDED USAGE

There is no RDI for ginger.

Children
Administer only under the advice of a doctor or health practitioner.

Adults
Capsules
One 100-milligram capsule up to three times daily.
Tincture
Three drops in an 8-ounce glass of water.
Tea
For relieving nausea or motion sickness, one cup within fifteen minutes of the onset of symptoms.

CAUTION!

Ginger is generally safe for everyone. There are, however, exceptions. People with hypertension should avoid it. Women with a history of miscarriage should check with a health care practitioner before using it.

Weak ginger tea may be used to soothe colicky infants. When using ginger oil, children and pregnant women should take only a half dosage.

Some herbalists recommend soaking in a ginger bath to relieve body aches and pains; however, this may irritate sensitive mucus membranes.

Finally, be aware that ginger tincture comes in a strong and a weak form. Know what you are buying and follow dosage instructions accordingly.

GINGKO
(*Gingko biloba*)

Overall Rating . . . . *Recommended*

To arrest memory loss due to
Alzheimer's . . . . *Recommended*

To combat impotence: . . . . *Recommended*

For treating incontinence . . . . *Not Recommended*

In 1512, Spanish explorer Ponce de Leon sailed north from Puerto Rico to Florida in search of the Fountain of Youth. He may have had more success in his search for the elixir if he had extended his trip to China. That's where he could have found the ancient gingko tree, the leaves of which have been used by the Chinese for centuries to prolong youth and promote longevity.

As our bodies age, the flow of blood and oxygen to the brain becomes less efficient. This increasing lack of vital brain nourishment can contribute to problems common in the elderly, such as dementia, senility, memory loss, dizziness, headache, ringing in the ears, and stroke. Gingko leaves are thought to ease these symptoms by helping to increase the flow of blood and oxygen to the brain.

Gingko is most commonly used in an extract form known as GBE, or gingko biloba extract, although it can also be found in tea, tincture, and tablet form. When taken for at least three months, gingko may improve

- attention span and alertness
- circulation throughout the body

🐾 eyesight

🐾 hearing

Gingko biloba is also commonly used to combat impotence, says Michael Murray, N.D., author of *Encyclopedia of Natural Medicine*. By increasing the level of essential fatty acids (EFAs), supplementing with gingko may increase blood circulation to the penis.

When used to promote cardiovascular health, gingko is sometimes combined with other herbs such as linden, hawthorn, greater periwinkle, or limeflower. Gingko may also have strong antioxidant qualities (meaning that it may help prevent long-term cellular damage) and, in combination with garlic and ginseng, can be found as part of an herbal "multivitamin." This combination may be taken to promote general health and physical well-being.

That's not all. This herb with the silly-sounding name may also strengthen your heart and reduce fluid retention in your body, thus helping you expel that excess water weight.

The Chinese have also learned that the nut of the female gingko tree works as a good remedy for asthma and other respiratory ailments. Both the nuts and leaves of the gingko tree, also known as the maidenhair tree, contain a substance known as ginkgolides. Gingkolides are thought to help ease asthma, allergies, and coughing by counteracting the protein found in blood that triggers spasms in the body's airways.

Gingko may help with kidney dysfunction. If you're troubled by incontinence, take a decoction of gingko nuts, made by boiling the nuts, straining the liquid from them, diluting the liquid, and drinking it.

Finally, although gingko has been touted as an aid for improving memory, research results have been mixed. The more definitive studies show gingko to be an effective blood thinner and helpful in some cases of moderate to severe Alzheimer's. However, its effect on memory is not proven.

RECOMMENDED USAGE

There is no RDI for gingko.

Children
May be useful for attention deficit disorder in children, but this has not yet been proven. Administer only under the advice of a doctor or health practitioner.

Adults
Capsules
One 40-milligram capsule up to three times daily.
Tincture
Three drops in an 8-ounce glass of water three times daily.

 CAUTION!

Although gingko is generally thought to be safe at small doses, large amounts may cause diarrhea, headache, irritability, restlessness, and may, over a long period of time, be toxic. As the benefits of gingko may take several months to appear, it is important that the proper dosage be taken. Before taking gingko, consult your doctor or a qualified herbalist or naturopath to determine how much you should take. If you use gingko to help treat asthma, it is especially important that you consult your doctor to ensure that it will not interfere with your current treatment. And be careful: Touching gingko may cause mild dermatitis in some people.

GINSENG
(*Panax ginseng*)

Overall Rating . . . . *Recommended*

For increased energy . . . . *Recommended*

To boost immunity . . . . *Not Recommended*

Because the ginseng root sometimes resembles a human form, the Chinese have long believed that this yellowish brown gnarled root exerts a tremendous influence throughout the entire body. Used for thousands of years in China, ginseng became increasingly popular in the West during the eighteenth century. So powerful was ginseng thought to be and so universally beneficial that when plants were being classified and assigned Greek names, ginseng was given the name panax, or panacea, meaning "cure-all."

Twenty-two different plants go by the name ginseng, which can make it difficult to determine precisely which type of ginseng is being used. Four types of ginseng—Korean (or Chinese), American, Tienchi, and Siberian—are commonly used for medicinal purposes. Panax ginseng refers to Korean ginseng, while panax quinquefolius is American ginseng. These two plants are very similar and are generally what we think of when requesting ginseng from an herbalist.

Tienchi ginseng, or *Panax notoginseng,* is thought to benefit the heart and help stop bleeding when applied to cuts and wounds. Although pregnant women should avoid all types of ginseng, Tienchi ginseng may be especially harmful to a fetus.

Finally, Siberian ginseng, *Eleutherococcus senticosus,* while not a true ginseng, does come from the same family of plants. It shares many properties and uses with its Korean and American cousins. As it is a different plant, it will be referred to as Siberian ginseng. Korean and American ginseng will simply be referred to as ginseng.

Although most Westerners depend on drinking coffee—and lots of it—to keep them alert throughout the day, ginseng likewise has a stimulating and revitalizing effect on the body, without the side effects of caffeine. What happens, according to experts, is that the herb accelerates the release of hormones from the adrenal glands. The result? It may

- improve and normalize overall body functions
- counteract the impact of physical stress
- help the body adapt to mental stress
- boost immunity

So, whether you've had a series of bad days or are suffering from the debilitating effects of a chronic disease, small amounts of ginseng may be soothing, energizing, or strengthening—depending on what your body needs.

Because ginseng is a substance—known as an adaptogen— that reportedly rejuvenates the body, athletes might give it a try during training to help them increase endurance, build stamina, and raise their performance to a new level.

Physical benefits are only part of the ginseng story. Doctors of traditional Chinese medicine widely state that it also has a powerful effect on short-term memory and mental alertness by counteracting the gradual dulling of memory and alertness. So, if you need something to help improve concentration while at the same time provide the energy necessary to be at your mental best, forget the coffee! Reach for the ginseng!

And here's another reason to keep it on hand: a better sex life. That's right. No wonder the Chinese call it a cure-all!

While traditional Chinese medicine prescribes ginseng only for men, these days it's used by both men and women for its aphrodisiac qualities. The Chinese recommend an herb known as dong quai, or Chinese angelica, for women. Try a ½ teaspoon of ginseng tincture in a glass of juice each day, and let Cupid's arrows fly!

Ginseng may also benefit men specifically by increasing testosterone levels and helping to reduce an enlarged prostate. Women may benefit from the plant estrogens found in ginseng that may counteract some of the symptoms common during menopause. In fact, studies from both China and Great Britain emphasize the efficacy of ginseng for menopausal symptoms. It can also boost fertility but should not be used following conception. Other therapeutic benefits of ginseng include

* easing depression
* alleviating stress-triggered migraine headaches
* combating coughs
* reducing blood sugar levels in diabetics
* helping to raise low blood pressure

If you get on the ginseng bandwagon, bear in mind that small amounts are best. Ginseng is generally taken in powdered form mixed into herbal tea or even, when fighting a cold or a fever, into chicken or rice soup. For example, ⅛ teaspoon of ginseng powder in a cup of herbal tea can be used to combat hayfever and sinusitis, a cold, or a bad cough.

This same cup of tea with ⅛ teaspoon of ginseng in it can be used as a general revitalizing tonic for body and mind. Taken for a few days before and for a few days after a flight, a cup of ginseng tea may counteract jet lag. It can be found in root form and in capsules, tablets, and tincture. No matter what form of ginseng you use, seek the advice of an herbalist to determine the proper dosage, and don't take it for longer than two months at a time without a break.

Although Siberian ginseng is technically not the same as panax ginseng, they share many therapeutic properties. Like ginseng, Siberian ginseng is an adaptogen that acts on the adrenal glands and is believed to help the body counteract stress, stimulate memory and alertness, and enhance athletic performance. Siberian ginseng, being milder, is a good substitute for those who may find ginseng too strong. Some herbalists recommend that ginseng be used primarily by the elderly or debilitated, and Siberian ginseng by the young, healthy, and strong.

 ## RECOMMENDED USAGE

There is no RDI for ginseng.

Children
Not advised for children. Administer only under the advice of a doctor or health practitioner.

Adults
Capsules
Two 1,000-milligram capsules up to three times daily.
Tincture
Three drops in an 8-ounce glass of water three times daily.

Not advised for pregnant or lactating women.

CAUTION!

Ginseng can be taken safely for up to two months, followed by a two- to three-week break before taking it again. Because it is such a strong stimulant, don't drink coffee or tea while using it.

Ginseng is a powerful stimulant and is not suitable for children, pregnant women, and those with high blood pressure.

Ginseng can cause headaches in some people and should not be taken if you have diarrhea. These same precautions apply when using Siberian ginseng, although it is thought to be safe when given in a half dosage to children over five years of age.

Finally, ginseng can be easily adulterated. Buy it from a reputable source, and be aware that many commercial products bearing the name contain little or no ginseng and will probably not have any therapeutic effect.

GLUTAMINE AND GLUTAMIC ACID

Overall Rating . . . . *Recommended*

To treat digestive problems . . . . *Recommended*

For increasing memory . . . . *Not Recommended*

In the body, glutamine and glutamic acid are interchangeable forms of the same amino acid. Glutamine helps maintain proper function of the nervous system. In the past it was touted to increase one's IQ, prevent senility, and treat depression, but these benefits have not been substantiated. One of the places glutamine works hardest is the intestines. When we eat glutamine-rich foods, a portion of this amino acid shoots into the cells of our small intestine, where it keeps them working properly. People who suffer from digestive and intestinal problems such as Crohn's disease, colitis, peptic ulcers, and ileitis might benefit from glutamine supplements.

 RECOMMENDED USAGE

There is no RDI for glutamine and glutamic acid.

Children
Administer only under the advice of a doctor or health practitioner.

Adults

Capsules

One 100-milligram capsule up to three times daily.

 ## CAUTION!

Anyone allergic or intolerant to the food preservative monosodium glutamate (MSG), may have similar reactions to glutamine and glutamic acid. Even though the amino acids are very different from MSG, if you have this allergy, consult with a health care practitioner prior to using glutamine supplements.

GOLDENSEAL
(*Hydrastis canadensis*)

Overall Rating . . . . *Recommended*

For applying topically as an antiseptic. . . *Recommended*

For boosting the immune system . . . . . . *Not Recommended*

Aplant native to the northeast, southeast, and midwest United States, goldenseal was used for centuries by Native Americans, early settlers and pioneers, and those interested in natural healing. Today, this small, valuable herb with its distinctive yellow root and hairy stalk, topped by a single white blossom, is endangered in the wild. Goldenseal is a victim of its own popularity. Not only that, but as its popularity has risen in recent years, many of the claims made regarding the plant's benefits have been called into question, and many of the recommendations concerning its use are contradictory.

Generally, most herbalists agree that goldenseal is a useful localized antiseptic. You can apply it topically to treat infection, reduce swelling and discomfort, and stanch sores. For example, poison ivy, eczema, and other skin ailments may respond to a wash made of goldenseal powder and warm water or cider vinegar. An alternative treatment for poison ivy combines equal parts raw honey and powdered goldenseal. Spread this mixture over the rash, cover it with a gauze bandage, and change the dressing daily. Goldenseal mixed with myrrh and marigold may help sores heal, while goldenseal mixed with witch hazel may reduce itching.

Eyes, ears, or throat bothering you? Goldenseal may be just what you need. An eyewash of goldenseal powder, crushed fennel seed tea, and baking soda can be swabbed over closed eyelids to help soothe conjunctivitis (strain the seeds out first). A mixture of two to three drops of goldenseal tincture, tincture of myrrh, and warm water may be used to treat sore throat, canker sores, and tender gums, while ear infections may respond to eardrops made from goldenseal tincture and water. However, these drops should not be used if there is any indication the eardrum is perforated.

While antiseptic uses of goldenseal are fairly straightforward, things get a bit trickier when it comes to ingesting goldenseal. Goldenseal powder, by itself or combined with other herbs and put into capsules, has been used for everything from fighting hay fever and sinusitis to treating menopausal symptoms. Until recently, goldenseal was accepted as an immunity booster and was mixed with other herbs—especially echinacea—to help ward off flus and the common cold.

Goldenseal does, however, have powerful cleansing properties. Known as a "bitter," because of its taste, goldenseal interacts with the taste buds to stimulate the digestive system, increasing the secretion of bile from the liver and gallbladder and promoting bowel movements. But that means you really and truly have to taste the bitter stuff to move things along (sorry, pills won't do the trick).

If your bowels are fine, you can avoid the bitter taste if you simply want to stimulate the spleen or help cleanse the lymphatic system. Simply take the capsule form. Beware, however, that because the effects of goldenseal can be powerful, many herbalists recommend that it be ingested only with great care, or not at all.

RECOMMENDED USAGE

There is no RDI for goldenseal.

Children
Administer only under the advice of a doctor or health practitioner.

Adults
One 535-milligram capsule up to twice daily.
Topically
Apply as an ointment, gel, or poultice.

 CAUTION!

Many of the recommendations concerning the ingestion of goldenseal are contradictory. Some herbalists believe that ingestion is safe, while others limit their recommendation of goldenseal to external uses. Before using goldenseal, check with your doctor, naturopath, or a qualified herbalist.

Goldenseal is a powerful plant with potentially powerful effects. One of the active ingredients, hydrastine, influences circulation and muscle tone. People with hypoglycemia, heart problems, and high blood pressure should not use goldenseal. Nor should pregnant women or nursing mothers.

Large doses of goldenseal can make you very sick and may be toxic. Be mindful that hydrastine remains in the body and accumulates over time, so prolonged use of it should be avoided. As a general rule, don't take the herb longer than two months at a time, because it can upset the balance of healthy bacteria in the intestines and interfere with the manufacture of essential B vitamins in the colon. Using acidophilus (bacteria often found in live yogurt and frequently added to other dairy products) can help maintain a healthy intestinal balance.

Goldenseal should only be taken in dried or powdered form; eating the fresh plant can damage the body's mucus membranes. Finally, exercise some caution when purchasing powdered goldenseal to ensure it has not been adulterated. Because goldenseal is such a popular herb, there have been instances of other herbs being added to it. Goldenseal powder should smell sweet, like licorice. It should have a bitter taste and a yellow or green color.

GOTU KOLA
(*Centella asiatica*)

Overall Rating . . . . *Recommended*

To calm the mind . . . . *Recommended*

For healing wounds . . . . *Highly Recommended*

Unless you're from the tropics or have been working with herbs for some time, you probably haven't heard of gotu kola. No, it's not a member of an exotic bear family—but it may help you "grin and bear" whatever your fast-paced life may be demanding of you these days. That's because the flower of the gotu kola plant is used for relaxation and clarity of mind. Gotu kola tea, or tincture, can be mixed with good old chamomile to make a pleasant brew that might also relieve an upset stomach.

Feeling good and relaxing is one thing, but gotu kola is also believed to improve concentration. The herbal equivalent of taking a deep breath and calling a personal time out, gotu kola may help restore a bit of equanimity when you're feeling overwhelmed and need to focus on the more important things of life.

One amazing study on wound healing, reported in the *European Journal of Gynecology,* stated that the extract of gotu kola helped to promote healing after an episiotomy. In fact, the women given the herb immediately after the procedure reported faster healing and less pain than those who had been given drugs. However amazing the results, more research is needed to substantiate these preliminary findings.

RECOMMENDED USAGE

There is no RDI for gotu kola.

Children
Administer only under the advice of a doctor or health practitioner.

Adults
Capsules
One 450-milligram capsule up to three times daily.

 CAUTION!

Gotu kola isn't a commonly known herb, and because of its odd name, take care not to confuse it with ground kola (or cola) nuts, which are a source of caffeine and won't do any good to help you relax. Long-term or continuous use of gotu kola is not recommended. A general rule of thumb is that a two-to-three week break from gotu kola is necessary after taking it for four to five weeks. And since high doses of gotu kola can cause headaches and itching, don't exceed the recommended dosage.

GREEN-LIPPED
MUSSEL EXTRACT
(*Perna canalialus*)

Overall Rating . . . . *Recommended*

For easing muscle and joint pain . . . . *Recommended*

You probably won't ever want to kiss a green-lipped mussel—but then again, if you're one of the millions of people who suffer from arthritis, you might. That's because this marine animal native to New Zealand contains an ingredient that blocks the activity of certain enzymes contributing to such painful symptoms related to certain forms of arthritis as

- swelling
- joint pain
- inflammation
- limited mobility in joints or connective tissues

In fact, studies at the Glasgow Homeopathic Hospital in Scotland report that after giving severely arthritic patients green-lipped mussel extract, a significant percentage not only experienced less pain and stiffness, but it also "helped the patients' ability to cope with life and enhanced their general health."

This is important to know since one in seven people (two thirds of them women) acquires either osteoarthritis or rheumatoid arthritis. And it's also good to know that green-lipped mussel extract doesn't have side effects, whereas the nonsteroidal anti-inflammatory drugs (NSAID) prescribed by most doctors for arthritic pain can cause ulcers or gastritis (inflammation of the stomach). In fact, green-lipped mussel extract actually exhibits a tendency to protect the stomach lining.

The Scotland studies show that it doesn't matter how long you've had the condition, how much it's progressed, or how old you are—it works across the board. It also doesn't matter if you have osteoarthritis (a degenerative condition where the joint cartilage is dissolving, leaving bone to painfully rub against bone) or rheumatoid arthritis (an autoimmune condition which inflames the joint linings). Both types of arthritis respond well to this treatment.

 ## RECOMMENDED USAGE

There is no RDI for green-lipped mussel extract.

Children

Not advised for children. Administer only under the advice of a doctor or health practitioner.

Adults

Capsules
One 350-milligram capsule up to three times daily.
Tincture
Three drops in an 8-ounce glass of water three times daily.

You can find the freeze-dried capsules of this supplement at most health food stores. Start treatment by taking between three and five 350-milligram capsules a day with food. Be aware that it may take four to six weeks for results to surface. Like the creature it comes from, progress is slow but sure.

Once you experience positive results, reduce your intake to two capsules per day.

 CAUTION!

Although people who are allergic to seafood, and in particular shellfish, don't consistently exhibit an allergic reaction to green-lipped mussel extract, if you do have such an allergy, take the supplement in small doses to start with and monitor yourself for a reaction. If you do react, simply quit taking the supplement, and the reaction will most likely fade.

If you are pregnant or nursing, contact a health care professional before using.

HAWTHORN
(*Crataegus oxycantha*)

Overall Rating . . . . *Recommended*

For treating heart disease. . . . . *Recommended*

For easing insomnia . . . . *Not Recommended*

With its delicate red fruit, creamy blossoms, and shiny green leaves, the diminutive hawthorn is a grace note in the forest, a small-scale tree that adds detail to the landscape. Also known as mayflower or may blossom, the hawthorn flowers in May and bears fruit in the fall. Coming upon this wonderful tree at any time of year, however, may do the heart good. Literally.

Your local M.D. may not know it yet, but this pretty little herb is used extensively in Europe for the treatment of heart disease. That's because it dilates the coronary vessels and increases the flow of blood and oxygen to the heart. This may improve heart metabolism. At the same time, the biological components that color hawthorn berries dark red appear to have a relaxing effect on the heart muscle itself. The upshot of all of this? When used under a doctor's supervision, hawthorn is thought to

- reduce angina attacks
- regulate high and low blood pressure
- reduce serum cholesterol levels
- prevent the deposit and buildup of cholesterol in arteries

And if all that isn't enough good news, hawthorn may also facilitate the absorption of vitamin C, thus strengthening the body's blood vessels and possibly improving circulation.

Hawthorn can be used in many forms. Tea, tinctures, tablets, juice, syrup, and extract are available commercially. These treatments can be made from the berries, leaves, or flowers of the hawthorn tree. Hawthorn may be combined with yarrow, lime blossom, or mistletoe in tea to treat hypertension. Hawthorn tea may also be effective for easing insomnia. Hawthorn berries, along with other dark-red and blue berries such as cherries and blueberries, appear to have anti-inflammatory properties that may ease the symptoms of rheumatoid arthritis and osteoarthritis.

While most of the attention paid to hawthorn in the West has focused on its potential impact on the heart and circulatory system, hawthorn has long been used in the East to aid digestion. In China, both green and ripe berries are used to help alleviate the discomfort of indigestion and overeating, while dried or charred berries are often used to treat diarrhea. So, as you can see, there's more than one way to spell "relief."

 ## RECOMMENDED USAGE

There is no RDI for hawthorn.

Children
Administer only under the advice of a doctor or health practitioner.

Adults
Capsules
One 100-milligram capsule up to three times daily.

CAUTION!

Since our lives depend on a healthy, beating heart, diseases that affect it should never be treated lightly. Therefore, make sure you work with a health care practitioner if you intend on using hawthorn or any other herb for a heart condition.

While hawthorn is generally thought to be gentle, *it can be toxic in large doses*. Also, beware not to use it with the heart drugs digoxin or digitoxin. It is important to note that any potential relief from hawthorn will not be immediate. Hawthorn may take several months to show results.

IODINE

Overall Rating. . . . . *Highly Recommended*

For cell growth, oxygen use, and
nerve function . . . . *Highly Recommended*

For reproductive functioning . . . . *Highly Recommended*

For skin, nail, and hair growth . . . . . . *Recommended*

Ever have days when you feel sluggish, slightly dim-witted, and a bit chilly? Do you get constipated on occasion? We all experience those "low" days now and then. It's just part of our biology.

But if you experience these symptoms fairly often, and along with that you're gaining weight, have little interest in sex, or you and your partner are having trouble conceiving, you could be low on iodine. That's because two-thirds of our body's iodine is contained within the thyroid, and thyroid hormones regulate overall metabolism and body temperature. So if you don't have enough iodine, your thyroid won't be able to function properly.

The good news is that, these days, it's easy to replenish low iodine levels and, in fact, rare to have deficiencies, as a recent report from Johns Hopkins Medical School illustrates. In the United States, iodine is added to table salt (400 micrograms per teaspoon for "iodized" table salt), and chances are good that you put salt on some of your food. Because of that, supplements are not typically necessary, which means you probably enjoy the benefits of enough iodine without even trying to. Those benefits include proper

- cell growth and oxygen use
- reproductive capabilities
- nerve function
- skin, nail, and hair growth

Salt isn't the only source of an extra dose of iodine. If you're a seafood lover, you'll find enormous amounts in seaweed, although for most of us, shellfish—oysters, crab, lobster, and shrimp—is preferable. Iodine is also found in meat and dairy products from animals raised on grain or feed from iodine-rich soils. Another great option is sunflower seeds.

 RDI

Children
40–150 micrograms

Adults
25–50 years: 150 micrograms
50+ years: 150 micrograms

Since iodine deficiencies are rare, you may indeed have a problem with your thyroid if you regularly experience fatigue, cold feet and hands, and the other symptoms listed above. Low thyroid function is quite common, especially among women over forty, perhaps due to a woman's changing body during premenopause and menopause, speculates menopause specialist Susan Lark, M.D., author of *The Women's Health Companion.* No one knows the exact reason for this, but blood tests can determine if your thyroid is either underactive or overactive. Natural or synthetic forms of thyroid are readily available to help balance out the condition. Some herbal remedies can also assist in boosting thyroid function.

CAUTION!

Long ago, before iodine was added to salt, deficiencies were common. Among adults, the result was generally goiters, a swollen thyroid attempting to churn out more hormones. These days, eating too many foods known as goitrogens (such as spinach, strawberries, lettuce, peaches, radishes, rutabagas, and mustards) can inhibit normal iodine/thyroid function and cause goiters. Cooking the foods prevents this from occurring.

Pregnant women should talk to their OB-GYN about iodine supplementation. (Lack of iodine can cause a form of mental retardation called cretinism.)

Ingesting more than twenty-five times the RDI, or 1,000 micrograms a day, can cause acne or goiters.

If you are taking lithium and want to supplement your iodine, or if you have these symptoms of an overdose, contact your doctor or health care practitioner immediately: rash, headache, difficulty breathing, metallic taste in the mouth, fever, or diarrhea.

IRON

Overall Rating. . . . . *Highly Recommended*

To strengthen the immune system. . . . *Highly Recommended*

For metabolizing cholesterol. . . . . . . *Highly Recommended*

For treating anemia . . . . *Highly Recommended*

For good skin and tissue elasticity. . . . *Highly Recommended*

Most people know that iron is an important mineral in our bodies and that the term "iron-poor blood" indicates a problem. But they don't really know what that means. Try holding your breath for three minutes and you'll get an idea. That's because iron-poor blood is literally blood that is starved of oxygen—which means it can't function properly, just as you can't function properly if you don't get enough oxygen. How does this relationship work? Iron acts as a mechanism to fuel your cells with oxygen. So take a nice deep breath and keep on reading!

The majority of iron in your body is contained in hemoglobin. It's commonly understood that all you need is about a teaspoon of iron to carry out the all-important task of transporting oxygen from your lungs to your cells. Iron also acts as a coenzyme and co-protein to determine how energy is released, as well as promote chemical changes throughout your body. Once the iron penetrates your cells—every cell in your body contains it—then it can go to work. Adequate levels of iron are critical for

❧ healthy myoglobin (an iron-protein mixture), which feeds muscles when they are working hard

- an efficient immune system
- proper metabolization of cholesterol
- production of connective tissues
- production of hemoglobin (in bone marrow)
- treatment of anemia
- normal growth
- good skin tone

Studies from the world-famous Mayo Clinic in Rochester, Minnesota, show that iron-rich blood can also relieve menstrual pain, stimulate the immune system, enhance physical stamina and performance, and assist with learning disabilities.

So where do you get this champion of minerals? You may remember your mother pushing beef, chicken, lamb, or pork liver in front of you as a child and saying, "It's good for you. It's full of iron." She was right. But there are plenty of other foods that contain it. Chocolate, for instance! And in between the extremes of liver and chocolate, you can eat apricots, cheddar cheese, cooked soybeans, curry powder, dried figs, baked potatoes (with the skin), seaweed, molasses, cooked spinach or turnips, spaghetti or macaroni noodles, cereal, shellfish, green leafy vegetables, and nuts.

 ## RECOMMENDED USAGE

Experts vary about how much iron is required for optimum health. The following information indicates an average. If you have questions, contact your health care professional.

Children
10–18 milligrams

Women

25–50 years: 15–75 milligrams
50 + years: 10–50 milligrams

Men

25–50 years: 10–18 milligrams
50 + years: 10–18 milligrams

Even though the earth contains an enormous supply of the mineral, the most common nutritional deficiency in the world is of iron. That's because we only absorb about 10 percent of the iron we ingest—which means growing toddlers, weight-conscious women eating fewer than 2,000 calories a day, pregnant or menstruating women, vegetarians, and the elderly probably aren't getting enough. It's a good idea, therefore, to have your iron checked during routine physical exams, especially since iron-deficient symptoms often don't show up until years later.

If you are low in iron, you'll experience one or more of the following symptoms:

- anemia, including overall fatigue, headaches, shortness of breath
- higher susceptibility to infection, due to immune deficiencies
- excessive bleeding during menstruation (menorrhagia)
- shrinking of lymphatic tissues
- learning disabilities in children
- heart palpitations during exercise
- cracked lips or difficulty swallowing
- craving for salt

Ironically, some recent studies indicate that iron-poor blood can actually cause heavy menstrual periods. That's in contrast to the well-documented fact that heavy periods can cause iron deficiencies. Gets tricky, but just be mindful of either possibility if you bleed heavily most of the time.

Inadequate amounts of iron are one reason for deficiencies, while malabsorption is another. Excessive amounts of coffee, tea, or alcohol, and normal amounts of milk, zinc, and vitamin E can inhibit iron absorption. Avoid these substances when taking an iron supplement or attempting to boost your intake with iron-rich foods. Taking vitamin C helps absorb iron.

If you're going to supplement, it's important to take easy-to-absorb forms of iron. Animal sources are more readily absorbed than plant sources. Supplements with iron carbonyl, ferrous sulfate, or ferrous gluconate are the best-absorbed over-the-counter products.

CAUTION!

Our bodies are masterfully able to absorb only the amounts of iron they really need, but accidental overdoses, especially in children (it only takes 3 grams), *can be fatal.* In fact, *iron overdose is the leading cause of poisoning deaths in children.* Be sure to keep all vitamins or iron supplements out of a child's reach. In case of accident, call 911 immediately.

If you want to supplement your iron intake, consider the following: the intestines regulate how much iron is absorbed. People with intestinal problems may absorb too little or too much iron. This can lead to oxidation and the release of free radicals, which can lead to cancer or heart disease. Iron supplements can create intestinal infections and constipation. Not everyone can tolerate iron supplements.

Don't supplement if you have had blood transfusions (unless directed by your doctor), kidney disease, rheumatoid arthritis, peptic ulcer disease, intestinal disease, Hodgkin's disease, or hepatitis.

Symptoms of an overdose include: diarrhea with blood, nausea with blood, abdominal pain, chest pain, and chills.

Consult a health practitioner prior to supplementation if you are taking calcium, antacids, or large amounts of aspirin.

JUNIPER
(*Juniperus communis*)

Overall Recommendation . . . . *Recommended*

**To releive symptoms of asthma,
sinusitis, head colds, and the flu** . . . . *Recommended*

If you've ever spent time hiking through the high plateaus of the desert of the American Southwest, close your eyes for a moment and picture your surroundings. Chances are, in and among your visions of blue sky and red-rock canyons, you saw a juniper, or cedar, tree. The photogenic sentinel of the desert, the juniper is a short, pinelike tree with a twisted trunk and branches, covered with reddish-brown and gray berries. If you haven't seen a juniper tree in the wild, then it is almost certain you're familiar with the garden variety found in yards everywhere. Common to both is an aroma as fresh, clean, and astringent as a blast of cool night air.

Given the distinctive scent of juniper, it's not surprising that one of its primary uses is to ease the symptoms of asthma, sinusitis, head colds, and the flu. Mixing several drops of juniper oil with water in a vaporizer is thought to stimulate easier breathing and sinus drainage and could even get rid of those pesky airborne germs invading your room. Drinking hot juniper tea is also recommended for easing cold and flu symptoms and may actually speed recovery.

Juniper oil can be very soothing when used in a poultice or as a rub to combat the aches and pains of arthritis and rheumatism. Juniper tincture is recommended by some for bruises and swelling and can be used to help ease sunburn, eczema, and psoriasis. If you've had a rough day, drop a handful of juniper's needlelike leaves into a warm bath to relax and soothe tired muscles. Or if you are out hiking in juniper country and fall and cut yourself, apply several mashed berries to help staunch and disinfect the wound.

Juniper oil combines well with other essential oils, such as pine, rosemary, cypress, and lavender, and has both cleansing and relaxing aromatherapy properties. Native Americans utilized juniper in smudge pots for cleansing the mind and body and to impart tranquillity. See for yourself if this works by putting dried juniper, in combination with sage or sweetgrass, in a small bowl. After letting the mixture burn for a few moments, blow it out and allow the smoke to waft throughout the room. Inhaling won't intoxicate you, but you could feel a bit more relaxed and clear-headed. Studies conducted by the French company Tissarand found that the smell of juniper was not only relaxing but invigorating, too.

Taken internally, juniper is thought to boost the immune system and encourage the elimination of uric acid and bodily toxins. Juniper is a strong diuretic and may be useful in aiding recovery from cystitis and urinary tract infections. Other diuretic herbs, such as the root or leaf of dandelion, are gentler, though. Juniper may help aid digestion and is recommended for combating occasional bouts of gas.

Finally, a study conducted in Spain indicates that drinking juniper tea can help diabetics decrease insulin dependency. Bear in mind, however, that *juniper tea will not cure diabetes,* and that long-term (as long, and as short, as several weeks) and excessive consumption of juniper tea could lead to kidney damage. If you are diabetic, check with your doctor before taking juniper tea.

RECOMMENDED USAGE

There is no RDI for juniper.

Children
Administer only under the advice of a doctor or health practitioner.

Adults
Capsules
One 100-milligram capsule up to three times daily.
Tincture
Three drops in 8-ounce glass of water as needed.
Inhaler
As needed.

 CAUTION!

Pregnant women should avoid juniper in any form, since it can stimulate uterine contractions. If you are pregnant, your best bet is to check with your doctor before using any herb. Juniper has intense cleansing properties and is too strong for infants and young children and should not be given to them. While juniper may be of use in easing cystitis or urinary tract infections, people with inflamed kidneys or chronic kidney problems should not use juniper, as it can lead to further irritation of the kidneys and urinary tract.

KAVA
(*Piper methysticum*)

Overall Rating . . . . *Recommended*

For alleviating stress, nervousness,
and anxiety . . . . *Recommended*

Its botanical name means "intoxicating pepper," and it's no wonder this herb has intoxicated stressed-out America. This latest natural remedy for stress, nervousness, and anxiety was originally used in ceremonial drinks in the Pacific Islands and is celebrated today as a safe and effective remedy for frazzled nerves and overworked psyches.

Kava influences the emotional command center of the brain, producing both psychological and physical relaxation responses, according to a study conducted at the Virginia Commonwealth University in Richmond. In this study, those taking kava had an improved sense of well-being and marked reduction in nervousness and tension compared with those on a placebo.

 RECOMMENDED USAGE

There is no RDI for kava.

Children
Not advised for children. Administer only under the advice of a doctor or health practitioner.

Adults

One 425-milligram capsule up to three times daily. Do not take for more than three months without consulting your doctor.

 CAUTION!

Do not use if you are pregnant or breastfeeding, suffering from Parkinson's disease or depression, or are taking any medications that affect the central nervous system.

Side effects are rare but include mild stomach upset and a dry, itchy rash. If such symptoms occur, discontinue use.

KELP/BLADDERWRACK
(*Fucus vesiculosus*)

Overall Rating . . . . *Recommended*

For treating hypothyroidism caused by
iodine deficiency . . . . *Recommended*

Remember one of the joys of childhood, an afternoon spent at the beach, stomping on pieces of washed-up seaweed? There was that gratifying "pop-pop-pop" beneath your feet as the kelp nodes burst. While jumping on kelp was fun, you wouldn't think of eating it, would you? Well, now that you're an adult, think again: Seaweed is one of the most nutritious foods on earth.

You've heard of kelp and seaweed, but what about bladderwrack? That's the name of the kelp most often used medicinally, a name under which kelp products are often found.

Bladderwrack is a tremendous source of iodine, which is essential for a healthy body (see Iodine entry). In children, a lack of iodine can result in delayed mental development or retardation. In adults, a deficiency of iodine can lead to hypothyroidism, a condition resulting when the thyroid operates at too low a level. Symptoms of hypothyroidism include extreme fatigue and lethargy, weight gain, and development of a goiter. By providing necessary iodine, bladderwrack can help to build and maintain a healthy mind and body.

Because the iodine found in bladderwrack can help to regulate the thyroid, kelp is sometimes marketed as a weight-loss tool, and claims have been made that, when applied topically, it can help get rid of cellulite. While weight loss may result when bladderwrack is used to combat hypothyroidism, it is not thought to be an effective remedy for obesity or cellulite.

Taking bladderwrack tablets or tea made with tincture or powder several times each day, however, may be helpful as a general metabolic stimulant. Bladderwrack may also help if you have difficulty absorbing minerals due to poor digestion. And, it may even slow the progress of arthritis and hardening of the arteries in the elderly.

An easy way to take small amounts of powdered bladderwrack is to sprinkle the powder onto food in place of salt and pepper. Bladderwrack oil can also be added to a bath for pain relief and to soothe excessively dry skin.

 ## RECOMMENDED USAGE

There is no RDI for kelp.

Children
Administer only under the advice of a doctor or health practitioner.

Adults
Capsules
One 100-milligram capsule up to three times daily.

 ## CAUTION!

If you use bladderwrack to help treat hypothyroidism, do so under a health care practitioner's supervision. The same holds true if you have any thyroid dysfunction.

Those on a sodium-restricted diet should use bladderwrack with care. Kelp gathered from the beach should not be used medicinally, due to the risk of contamination.

KOMBUCHA MUSHROOM

Overall Rating . . . . *Not Recommended*

For treating autoimmune disorders,

including AIDS . . . . *Not Recommended*

We pitch them in a stir-fry. We pick them fresh from forests and present them as gourmet fare. Some people eat them for their hallucinogenic insights, while others throw festivals to celebrate their mystery and beauty. So why shouldn't there be a mushroom from which we concoct a tea and glean essential nutrients?

There is no scientific evidence to prove what some people exuberantly proclaim about the medicinal properties of kombucha mushroom. But the liquid gathered from a fermented mushroom does, in fact, contain glucuronic acid, lactic acid, vitamins, amino acids, and antibiotic substances. And all those are good for you.

First grown and utilized in eastern Asia, the unique benefits of drinking a tea from the fermented kombucha mushroom soon made their way to Europe and the Americas. Now, people in all corners of the planet claim that the mushroom's unusual blend of bacteria and yeast can relieve symptoms of a wide range of autoimmune disorders. Perhaps the most significant claim is that it has antiviral properties and can reverse the symptoms of AIDS.

While studies do not support either beneficial effects nor adverse side effects, a 1997 journal article researched by the Texas Health Sciences Center indicated that some people may experience gastrointestinal toxicity after consuming the tea. The symptoms observed were allergic reaction, jaundice, nausea, vomiting, and head and neck pain.

 RECOMMENDED USAGE

There is no RDI for kombucha mushroom.

Children
Not advised for children. Administer only under the advice of a doctor or health practitioner.

Adults
Capsules
One 100-milligram capsule up to three times daily.
Tincture
Three drops in an 8-ounce glass of water three times daily.

 CAUTION!

Some people think home-growing the mushroom provides opportunities for bad bacteria to enter the liquid. Others claim that the properties inherent to the mushroom repel bad bacteria. Grow this mushroom and drink its liquid *at your own risk* and be sure that you trust the source from which you acquired the original culture.

LADY'S MANTLE
(*Alchemilla vulgaris*)

Overall Rating. . . . . *Recommended*

For treating gynecological problems . . . . *Recommended*

For women who are tired of gulping down over-the-counter meds for menstrual pain, heavy bleeding, or irregular cycles, lady's mantle might be just what the doctor—or herbalist—orders. For reasons science hasn't yet been able to spell out, lady's mantle can actually help regulate menstrual cycles and ease cramps, while its astringent qualities successfully reduce heavy bleeding.

Before "modern" medicine took over, lady's mantle was widely used to treat most gynecological problems, as well as dress wartime wounds. It was, in fact, considered a bit of magic (its Latin name, "Alchemilla" means magic) for producing the grand results it did. While studies have yet to prove its efficacy, long-time effective use in home remedies has shown it to be a useful supplement when used carefully.

For women whose doctors don't know why they can't get pregnant, lady's mantle is thought to be helpful for infertility. It's considered a great toner and strengthener for the uterus. But once you are pregnant, stop using it immediately, as it stimulates the uterus and could bring on premature labor.

RECOMMENDED USAGE

There is no RDI for lady's mantle.

Children
Not advised for children. Administer only under the advice of a doctor or health practitioner.

Adults
This herb is widely available in health food stores and can be found as a tea, tincture, or ointment.

To treat menstrual cramps, drink the tea in combination with marigold. For excessive bleeding or irregular periods, use it with yarrow.

To make the tea, place 1 or 2 teaspoons of the leaves in hot water. Drink the tea up to five times per day.

The tincture is also good for menstrual cramps.

To treat vaginal itch, combine 50 grams of lady's mantle ointment, 15 milliliters of the tincture, and 20 milliliters of rosewater. This can be used as a douche or salve.

 CAUTION!

Avoid lady's mantle if you are pregnant.

LAVENDER
(*Lavandula officinalis*)

Overall Rating. . . . . *Recommended*

For cleaning and healing burns. . . . . . *Recommended*

For relieving stress . . . . *Highly Recommended*

Whether lavender makes you think of English sachets and soap or a breezy, sun-baked day on a hillside in Provence, the scent of this herb is evocative. A common component of perfume, as well as an ingredient used to balance many essential oils, lavender has an uplifting and soothing scent. Used in the bath, as a massage oil, or as an inhalant, the herb is a traditional remedy for stress, depression, headaches, and insomnia. Yet its uses go far beyond traditional aromatherapy.

Lavender flower tea, especially when combined with topical application of lavender oil, may give an extra boost to your fight against stresses of all kinds. Its taste may remind you of your grandmother's soap, but lavender does contain natural sedatives and components that slow nerve impulses to help you relax. Lavender may therefore help lower high blood pressure. Most of our information on lavender is anecdotal, but given its long-standing use, we have recommended it for select purposes.

Did you overdo it on the tennis court or in the garden last weekend? A lavender oil massage or a bath scented with lavender flowers may help soothe your tired muscles. If you have a cranky baby, lavender oil may help cool fiery diaper rash, while very weak lavender tea is an old-time remedy for colic. Lavender flowers added to brandy or rum may help ease a nasty cough, as may lavender tea. You might also want to try rubbing your chest with lavender oil to help break up congestion.

Lavender contains a natural antiseptic that may be helpful when used as a tea to

- wash burns, insect bites, and stings
- clean cuts
- soothe sunburn
- treat cold sores

Other less common uses of lavender include

- mixing with chamomile and marigold tea to recover from childbirth
- rinsing hair with lavender oil and water to get rid of lice and nits
- washing the mouth with lavender tea to banish bad breath

Finally, lavender is thought to be an effective natural insect repellent and an aphrodisiac. Looking for a picturesque, bug-free location for a romantic picnic? Picture a sun-swept purple hillside overlooking the Mediterranean. The scent of lavender is in the air . . . and if bugs are a nusance, pull out the lavender oil!

 RECOMMENDED USAGE

There is no RDI for lavender.

If you are making your own oils or tea, use 1 teaspoon flowers per pint of water or two drops of oil per one cup of carrier oil (olive or vitamin E oil, for example).

To treat headaches and depression, take no more than 5 milliliters of the tincture twice daily.

To relieve sunburn, add several drops of lavender oil to water and gently apply to affected area. In an undiluted form, the oil can also be used to repel insects.

To ease symptoms of respiratory discomforts, combine 1 milliliter of oil with five drops of chamomile oil, and add to 10 milliliters of carrier oil.

 CAUTION!

Lavender *oil* is toxic when taken internally. Even when used externally, it should be used sparingly. Lavender can stimulate the uterus and is not recommended for pregnant women. Consult with your doctor before giving even a weak tea to your baby. A half dose is recommended for children. People with low blood pressure are advised to avoid lavender. Finally, if you are looking to relax, avoid Spanish lavender—it's a stimulant!

LECITHIN

Overall Rating . . . . *Highly Recommended*

To improve mental functioning . . . . . . *Highly Recommended*

To improve liver functioning . . . . *Highly Recommended*

For reducing cholesterol . . . . *Highly Recommended*

Lecithin is a natural source of choline, the B complex responsible for our ability to connect our feelings to our behaviors. It also binds our cell membranes together.

A common use for lecithin is to thicken foods like mayonnaise and ice cream. And even though mayonaise contributes to a good tuna sandwich and ice cream is a relief on a hot afternoon, there are many more benefits to lecithin.

Lecithin is also thought to be helpful in treating neurological problems, including developmental disabilities, manic depression, Alzheimer's disease, and tardive dyskinesia. In fact, some preliminary studies using therapeutic dosages of phosphatidylcholine (the key component of lethicin) showed improved memory in both normal and Alzheimer's patients. These studies, however, did not conclusively assess target dosage zones and long-term results. However, if Alzheimer's is a concern, a dosage of 15 to 30 grams of phosphatidylcholine may be tried daily, for up to two weeks. Any improvement will be noticeable during this time period.

Lethicin also may

🐾 lower cholesterol and keep arteries clean and healthy
🐾 assist with fat metabolism

❧ possibly preserve the integrity of nerve coverings in people with multiple sclerosis

Lecithin could help justify eating more of that ice cream on hot afternoons, since it may actually help you lose weight. The soy form of lecithin, known as soya lecithin, helps your body break up and metabolize fat, using it up so that it doesn't stay parked on your thighs.

It's easy to get enough lecithin from your diet, since it's in a variety of foods. Animal sources rich in lecithin include caviar, egg yolk, liver, milk, and muscle meats. Good vegetable sources are cabbage, cauliflower, chickpeas, green beans, lentils, rice, soybeans, and split peas.

Lecithin supplements are available, but because lecithin is hailed as a natural form of choline, it may be best to get it through foods. Beware, however, that if you're taking nicotinic acid along with lecithin, it will decrease lecithin's capabilities.

 ## RECOMMENDED USAGE

There is no RDI for lethicin.

Children
Administer only under the advice of a doctor or health practitioner.

Adults
Capsules
One 100-milligram capsule up to three times daily.

CAUTION!

Few people need lecithin supplements, as we get plenty of it in our diet without trying. If you do supplement, it's possible to get too much lecithin, resulting in nausea, vomiting, dizziness, and depression. If you have any of these symptoms, stop taking the supplements and contact a physician.

People with enzyme deficiencies who take lecithin may end up with fishy-smelling breath and skin. Speak to a health care practitioner about this. Also, Alzheimer's patients taking lecithin supplements are more likely to suffer from stomach upset. If this is the case, they should discontinue use.

LEMON BALM
(*Melissa officinalis*)

Overall Rating . . . . *Recommended*

For treating herpes simplex . . . . *Recommended*

To alleviate stress and headaches . . . . *Recommended*

A relative of the mint plant, lemon balm seems like the perfect addition to a tall glass of iced tea: lemony and minty all in one. In fact, lemon balm is easily grown and can be added to lots of different foods to uplift the cook and excite the palate. Not only will your homemade culinary achievements taste delicious, but you'll feel good, too, as lemon balm is thought to promote digestion and ward off gas.

Also known as bee balm because the fuzzy insects just can't resist it, lemon balm contains components called terpenes that calm and relax the body's central nervous system. Terpenes help with digestion and may also

- combat insomnia and nightmares
- ease migraines and tension headaches
- fight depression
- calm heart palpitations and irregular heart beat
- soothe eczema, shingles, and other skin diseases related to stress
- relax teething and colicky babies

One of the most common uses for lemon balm is to apply topically to treat herpes simplex in the mouth. This is because the antiviral properties that make up the supplement seem to work together to prevent the virus from further infecting other cells—and is much more effective than any sole chemical. In fact, a comprehensive series of trials from three German hospitals and a dermatology center showed that when lemon balm was used topically upon the first sign of cold sores, patients were able to limit the cold sores to the initial breakout.

Therapeutic doses of lemon balm can also be consumed as a tea; massaged into the back, head, and neck to relieve stress; added to a bath; or washed over problem skin, depending on the condition you wish to treat.

 ## RECOMMENDED USAGE

There is no RDI for lemon balm.

Children

Not advised internally for children. Administer topically only on the advice of a doctor or health practitioner.

Adults

For herpes simplex (cold sores on the mouth, *not* genital herpes), apply lemon balm immediately upon first sign of breakout.

If you are suffering from a cold, lemon balm tea may help break a fever. Because lemon balm contains polyphenols that combat viruses and infections, lemon balm tea used as a drink or a wash may also help clean cuts, heal cold sores, reduce acne, and fight herpes infections. You may relieve asthma or upper respiratory infections by rubbing lemon balm ointment into your chest or inhaling its steam from a cup of tea. A nice moist lemon balm facial could do double duty: cleansing your pores and soothing your lungs at the same time!

If PMS or menstrual cramps are causing you trouble, lemon balm tea may calm and ease your symptoms, while helping to regulate your monthly cycle.

Finally, lemon balm is a natural insect repellent. Simply add 5 milliliters of lemon balm oil to 100 grams of ointment base and apply generously to your skin. If you are camping out among the mosquitoes and gnats, try burning some lemon balm leaves in your campfire to repel those flying pests, or rub your picnic table with lemon balm ointment to keep the creepy-crawlies away. But be fore-warned: While you may fight off the mosquitoes, you are extending an open invitation to honeybees—they find this balm irresistible!

 CAUTION!

Culinary uses are generally safe for pregnant women. Fresh lemon balm is much more effective than dried lemon balm.

LICORICE
(*Glycyrrhiza glabra*)

Overall Rating. . . . . *Highly Recommended*

For treating digestive disorders . . . . . . *Highly Recommended*

To boost energy . . . . *Highly Recommended*

For treating autoimmune disorders . . . *Recommended*

Before the myriad assortment of candies splashed store shelves, there were just a few tried-and-true goodies that kids (and adults) depended on to satisfy a sweet tooth. Chewy, ropelike licorice was one of them. Actually, though, store-bought candies are generally flavored with anise, not licorice. So the truth is, Americans have very little experience with the real substance, including its wide range of medicinal properties and uses.

Oddly, licorice is a root from a legume. We grow it here, in small pockets of the United States, but it's indigenous to southern and central Europe and to Asia. Called "the grandfather of all herbs" by the Chinese, this is the most-used herb in Chinese medicine. Very often, the Chinese use it to sweeten or balance the use of other herbs. Chinese medicine has turned to licorice for hundreds of years to combat a variety of ailments.

More recently, both the British and Japanese have studied it and found conclusive evidence that backs up what the Chinese have always claimed: Licorice is an excellent treatment for stomach upsets, especially duodenal and peptic ulcers. In fact, the British medical journal *Lancet* maintains that deglycyrrhizinated licorice (DGL) is more effective than over-the-counter or prescription drugs to treat, heal, and prevent reoccurrence of duodenal ulcers. And unlike drug treatments, DGL poses no side effects.

The difference between regular licorice and DGL is simple: Raw licorice contains glycyrrhetinic acid and DGL doesn't. And although glycyrrhetinic acid just might prevent cavities, in large doses it absolutely *raises* blood pressure. Consequently, DGL is the preferred form of licorice for long-term treatments.

There are (at least) two remarkable qualities of licorice. First, the properties that make up the licorice plant are effective in dealing with ulcers. Second, when drunk as a tea or taken in capsule form, licorice produces a protective lining around the stomach and small intestines that essentially wards off the intrusion of any unpleasant acids. That's why it's good for ulcers and indigestion. It has also been used throughout the years to treat a variety of conditions, including gastrointestinal symptoms (especially pain related to gas), high cholesterol, sore throats, allergies, arthritis, low energy levels, chest coughs and bronchitis, hypoglycemia, heart palpitations, and mental instability.

Licorice contains triterpenoids and phenolics, known cancer-fighting agents. In fact, licorice is now being studied to determine if it could be used to treat some cancers.

According to research conducted in Tokyo at the Oriental Medicine Research Center and reported in the medical journal *Herbal Gram,* licorice also contains potent antiviral properties that might effectively treat autoimmune diseases such as lupus, Addison's disease, Parkinson's disease, and Graves' disease.

 RECOMMENDED USAGE

There is no RDI for licorice.

You can find licorice in any health food store in the form of tea or capsules or as the raw root.

If you have a duodenal ulcer, drink at least two cups of tea per day, or if your symptoms are very serious and you're considering surgery, first try taking up to 4.5 grams of DGL per day for up to six weeks. This has provided great relief for those suffering from the most severe ulcers.

Drink licorice tea or use a decoction or tincture to treat coughs and chest pain.

To rid yourself of irritating stomach acids, take 5 grams of powder in water for up to two weeks.

If gas pain is bothering you, chew 380 to 500 milligrams of licorice twenty minutes before eating. Take some peony or chamomile with the licorice, and the results may be even better.

Since licorice is fifty times sweeter than sucrose, you can sweeten other, less appetizing teas with it. Mix it with ginseng tea for a good energy booster.

You can make a poultice by simmering the root with flaxseed, then apply to swollen joints or nonmalignant growths. Or buy a cream or paste to treat psoriasis.

Licorice is safe for kids, too. To ease their sore throats, coughs, or chest irritations, hand them sticks of the root to suck on. They'll like the flavor, and it will help.

 CAUTION!

Extended use of raw licorice can raise blood pressure. *Don't use it if you already have high blood pressure.* Excessive use can cause diarrhea. Don't use licorice if you are on any drugs containing digoxin.

LYSINE

Overall Rating . . . . *Recommended*

For treating herpes simplex 1 & 2 . . . *Recommended*

To heal damaged tissues and
encourage bone growth . . . . *Highly Recommended*

Since your body is always working—all the time, twenty-four hours a day, every breathing moment—that means it's always rebuilding itself. Yes, it's wise to be mindful of what you eat and of what foods or supplements can assist with physical challenges you may have. But, for the most part, your bones, hair, skin, and red blood cells rebuild themselves without you having to do much of anything.

Amino acids are largely the reason why. Lysine is one of the essential amino acids that enable you to go about your daily life, completely unaware of the construction work taking place within you around the clock. Ironically, however, lysine is one of eight essential amino acids your body does not manufacture on its own. You have to eat certain foods to obtain adequate amounts of it. In turn, once joined up with the other aminos, it goes about its job of rebuilding you.

Specifically, lysine is thought to:

- encourage bone growth
- utilize fatty acids
- produce antibodies, hormones, and enzymes
- heal damaged tissue
- contribute to the formation of collagen

Lysine has gained slightly more notoriety than the other amino acids because, in addition to doing all the things already listed, experts believe it successfully treats some really uncomfortable conditions. Most notably, herpes simplex 1 (usually manifested as cold sores or canker sores on the lips or in the mouth or throat) and herpes simplex 2 (realized as genital sores). Gulping down 2,000 to 3,000 milligrams of the supplement at the first sign of an outbreak can reduce the intensity of it or ward it off completely. How? Because lysine apparently intercepts the ability of another amino acid, arginine, from feeding the herpes virus.

Taking lysine for herpes isn't a scientifically proven treatment, but ask one of the 500,000 people who get herpes every year if it works, and many of them will say that it does. It is this wealth of anecdotal evidence that supports our recommendation.

For those suffering from heart disease, taking 3,000 milligrams per day can relieve pain from angina both before and after bypass surgery. Other claims give lysine credit for lowering high blood pressure, solving certain fertility problems, decreasing triglyceride levels, enabling the body to use calcium more efficiently, improving concentration, and keeping skin younger looking. But again, these are anecdotal reports; no scientific substantiation exists.

 RECOMMENDED USAGE

There is no RDI for lysine.

Children
Not advised for children. Administer only under the advice of a doctor or health practitioner.

Adults

Capsules

One 1,500-milligram capsule up to three times daily.

Tincture

Three drops in an 8-ounce glass of water three times daily.

Even though we know we need lysine, it's difficult to determine exactly how much is necessary. Again, since deficiencies are uncommon, it's safe to say that most people get enough. Even so, some experts believe that we need about 7 milligrams per pound of body weight.

For herpes, take 2,500 to 3,000 milligrams at the first sign of outbreak.

 CAUTION!

Rare deficiencies can be spotted, with symptoms of fatigue, red eyes, dizziness, inability to concentrate, and anemia.

Don't take lysine supplements if you are diabetic or have blood sugar problems. Never give them to children, as they may retard growth.

MAGNESIUM

Overall Rating . . . . *Highly Recommended*

To strengthen the
cardiovascular system . . . . *Highly Recommended*

For relieving migraines . . . . *Recommended*

For building strong bones . . . . *Highly Recommended*

For treating asthma . . . . *Recommended*

For relieving PMS . . . . *Recommended*

When our predecessors first swam up out of the bubbling broth known as the primordial ocean, they weren't swimming in salt water. Back then, water was filled with magnesium and potassium. Considering how important magnesium is to our bodies, it's not surprising that it's been with us all along. This essential mineral pushes every single one of our enzymes into action and is necessary for the functioning of our cells. The important processes in which magnesium plays a major role include

* regulating the metabolism and promoting healthy nerve function
* strengthening the cardiovascular system
* helping bones grow and keeping teeth rich in calcium
* producing insulin and helping diabetics maintain healthy blood sugar levels
* relaxing muscles after they've been contracted

Magnesium may also be helpful in subduing mental disturbances such as schizophrenia, delirium, confusion, and convulsions;

ensuring healthy pregnancies; and preventing the recurrence of kidney stones.

Magnesium works especially hard to keep our cardiovascular system in peak condition. Teaming up with calcium and the electrolytes, it builds up blood vessels so they're flexible and strong. To that end, and as a natural muscle relaxant, magnesium relieves people who suffer from angina, a condition in which an artery supplying blood to the heart goes into a painful spasm. Similarly, it can help relieve migraine headaches—also vascular—especially when they occur as part of a woman's menstrual cycle, recent reports from Europe are indicating. While supplementation did not affect the occurrence of migraines, almost 30 percent of the people in the study who took magnesium supplements claimed relief from the headaches they had.

And anyone suffering from asthma knows how frightening it can be when bronchial tubes close up and prevent air from getting to the lungs. Magnesium's relaxing properties can help open airways and bring the asthma attack to a halt.

The list goes on: It helps keep blood pressure low and steady, and it can alleviate symptoms of premenstrual syndrome. Women suffering from moodiness, headache pain, and tender breasts may find relief with magnesium supplements.

If you trust the water from your tap, and it's considered "hard" water, you can get magnesium just from drinking a glass of that water. Animal sources of this mineral include milk, cheese, and different meats and seafoods—particularly flounder. Plant and vegetable sources include oatmeal, rice, almonds, cashews, peanuts, black beans, soybeans and limas, bananas, broccoli, potatoes baked with the skin, figs, and molasses.

RDI

Children
Administer only under the advice of a doctor or health practitioner.

Adults
25+ years: 400 milligrams

There is no RDI for children, but experts agree that daily intake of 80 to 360 milligrams is appropriate for children one year old to twenty-five years. Check with your pediatrician for specific dosage recommendations.

Magnesium supplements come in a wide variety. Magnesium carbonate and magnesium oxide are often recommended because they contain the highest concentrations. Magnesium aspartate and magnesium glycinate are also good because they're easier to absorb.

Magnesium is most beneficial when taken with calcium, and nutritionists suggest a calcium-magnesium ratio of 1 to 1 or 1 to 1.5.

 CAUTION!

Signs of low magnesium include emotional agitation, such as confusion, tension, and irritability, and muscle disturbances, such as irregular heartbeat, tremors, cramps, and the sensation that your extremities are "asleep." Diarrhea and vomiting may also occur.

Deficiencies tend to occur in people with inadequate diets, including alcoholics, anorexics, bulimics, and diabetics. People with stomach or intestinal conditions that impair their ability to properly digest food may also be low in magnesium. Diuretics and birth control pills inhibit our ability to absorb the mineral.

Magnesium is nontoxic, even when taken in large doses. *Nutritional supplements and antacids containing magnesium can, however, be highly toxic for people with kidney failure or congestive heart failure.* If you have one of these conditions, seek the advice of a physician prior to supplementation.

MA HUANG
(*Ephedra sinica*)

Overall Rating . . . . *Not Recommended*

To treat respiratory conditions. . . . . *Not Recommended*
For combating colds, flus, and fever. . . . *Not Recommended*

Some things never change.

Five thousand years ago, the Chinese sought out this desert shrub to help with a variety of respiratory ailments and—for whatever reason—to promote sweating. That's because ma huang contains a powerful medicinal property known as ephedrine.

These days, Americans reach for such popular over-the-counter drugs as Sudafed, Actifed, and Contact to treat respiratory irritations due to the common cold. That's because these drugs are full of the synthetic form of ephedrine. Still effective after all these years.

It was, however, the Chinese in 1924 who actually isolated ephedrine from the ma huang plant, identifying it as the healing agent. A few short years later, American pharmaceutical companies recognized its overwhelming benefits and began to produce the synthetic version.

Regardless of whether you harvest your own ma huang or jaunt down to the nearest drug store for the synthetic version, the effects of ephedrine and psuedoephedrine are powerful and effective for the treatment of bronchitis, asthma, hay fever, wheezing, whooping cough, and labored breathing.

What's more, ma huang promotes sweating and so can be used to combat colds, flu, and fever. It's also a natural diuretic and works well to treat water retention.

There are several American-grown versions of ma huang, and although they contain far less ephedrine and so are less potent, they can still be used for their medicinal properties. You can find them under the names Mormon tea, squaw tea, cowboy tea, popotillio, and desert herb.

Some people have found ma huang an effective agent for weight loss, especially in conjunction with green tea and cola nut. It's true that the combination of these herbs increases the metabolic rate of the breakdown of fat. But herbalists are shying away from these combinations since they have been known to cause heart attacks and damage the nervous system. In fact, the sudden death of a healthy college student in 1997 was attributed to ma huang, reported the *Journal of Clinical Psychopharmacology*. The student had consumed a ma huang–containing drink and died several hours later of ephedrine toxicity. Some health care practitioners advise against using green tea and cola nut at all while taking ma huang. The risks are too serious.

 RDI

There is no RDI for ma huang.

This powerful herb is available in a powder form, tincture, and decoction.

To treat asthma, chills, and hay fever, take 1 to 4 milliliters of the tincture three times a day.

For colds, coughs, asthma, and hay fever, put 1 to 2 teaspoons of the herb in water, boil the water, and then simmer for fifteen minutes. Drink up to three cups a day, with food, for short-term use only. Don't consume coffee or tea while utilizing this therapy.

 CAUTION!

This herb is so potent that some states in this country are making moves to outlaw the over-the-counter sale and use of ma huang, the original and rawest form of ephedrine. Seem extreme? Perhaps not. Ephedrine is a lot like adrenaline and can cause some pretty extreme reactions: increased blood pressure, heart attacks, damage to the nervous system, uncontrolled sweating, increased blood flow to the brain.

Don't use this herb without the guidance of a doctor or health care provider, and certainly don't use it if you have heart disease or high blood pressure; if you're weak, insomniac, nervous, or have poor digestion; or if you perspire a lot.

MANGANESE

Overall Rating. . . . . *Highly Recommended*

To build strong bones and tissue. . . . . *Highly Recommended*

To strengthen the immune system. . . . *Highly Recommended*

To increase energy level . . . . *Highly Recommended*

There seems to be a common reaction to the enigmatic mineral known as manganese: a befuddled expression, scratching of the head, and asking "What is this?" That's because this mysterious substance (not to be confused with magnesium) is essential for life, yet we know very little about it. From the bits and pieces that have been gleaned, manganese seems to have its hand in quite a few pots. Its primary functions include

- development of bone and connective tissue
- proper nerve function
- support of the immune system
- energy production

Much like calcium, manganese helps bones grow. When we break a bone or tear a muscle or ligament, manganese fixes us up by helping fuse bones back together, building new connective tissue, and clotting our blood. Related to these functions, it has been proven to improve our muscle reflexes. Manganese may even fight osteoporosis, which weakens the bones in older age.

The worrisome or absentminded may want to use this mineral, as manganese works in the nervous system to keep nerves functioning smoothly. It's still unclear whether or not it improves memory, but manganese has been shown in some clinical instances to prevent seizures, which may benefit epileptics—though this hasn't been conclusively proven. Manganese is also vital to the production of dopamine, a neurotransmitter that sends messages to the brain, as well as thyroxin, an important hormone secreted by the pituitary gland. These functions are significant for healthy function of the central nervous system as well as for reproduction.

This industrious mineral also supports the immune system, where it's an essential ingredient to one of our body's most powerful antioxidants: superoxide dismutase (SOD). In fact, some experts think manganese may be an antioxidant in its own right. Manganese acts like a capable general by inspiring our antibodies and other fighter cells to protect the body from invasions by viruses, bacteria, and other pathogens.

On a metabolic level, manganese is critical for the synthesis of fat, protein, and carbohydrates. It helps distribute glucose throughout the body and regulates blood sugar levels. Because of this ability, some diabetics are now seeking the benefits of manganese to control their blood sugar. Much the way it activates our antibodies, manganese stimulates the enzymes that help nutrients such as vitamin B_1, vitamin C, and biotin perform their functions. As a happy benefit of all of this stimulation, manganese may increase our overall energy level.

Studies from the United Kingdom show that folks there get nearly half their manganese from drinking tea, reports *Nutrition*. This nutrient can also be found in nuts, fruits, and vegetables—especially avocados, blueberries, beans, broccoli, chestnuts, hazelnuts, pecans, pineapples, peas, seaweed, and spinach. Beans and whole grains are sources of manganese as well, but they contain fiber and phytic acid, which prevent the body from absorbing this substance. Actually, getting manganese from food tends to be generally hampered by poor absorption. Supplements may be a better choice.

RDI

Children
1–5 milligrams

Adults
25+ years: 2 milligrams

New information about manganese continues to surface, so the current RDI is considered extremely conservative.

When shopping for a manganese supplement, two of the best choices are manganese sulfate and manganese gluconate. While the sulfate tends to be a tad less pricey, the gluconate is a bit easier to digest. Both forms do the trick, however, so which one you choose is simply a matter of preference.

 CAUTION!

Manganese will interact with other substances. Taking excessive amounts of manganese may prevent our body from absorbing the iron it needs. Conversely, a lot of calcium, magnesium, and phosphate may inhibit our absorption of manganese. Women using birth control pills may want to consider manganese supplementation, since oral contraceptives prevent the body from utilizing the mineral.

If you get your manganese through foods and vitamin supplements, the risk of toxicity is minimal. Adverse reactions may include lack of appetite, headaches, fatigue, cramping in the legs, and trouble breathing. If you encounter these symptoms, discontinue use and contact your health practitioner.

There have been cases in Chile where miners who inhaled

manganese dust exhibited a kind of manganese madness. Known as *locura manganica,* this condition is extremely dangerous, inciting mania, depression, and convulsions. But unless you work in an environment where manganese dust is prevalent, you aren't at high risk.

MELATONIN

Overall Rating . . . . *Recommended*

For treating sleep disorders . . . . *Recommended*

To promote longevity . . . . *Recommended*

To reduce seasonal affective disorder . . . *Recommended*

To reduce cluster headaches. . . . . *Not Recommended*

For preventing jet lag . . . . *Recommended*

I t's one of the best sensations around. In the darkness of the bedroom, snug under the covers, muscles slowly melt into weightlessness. The drift from real time to dream time begins, and life in slumber land slips us into another dimension.

We couldn't go to that other dimension without our internal clock, or circadian rhythm. This unique clock keeps time by the metaphoric battery of the pineal gland, that tiny organ tucked deep in our brains. When it gets dark outside, the pineal gland secretes the hormone melatonin, which in a slow fade makes us sleepy—and provides us with that magical transition from the waking to the sleeping state.

Taking melatonin supplements may help with the insomnia we all experience on occasion. It can be even more beneficial for those who travel frequently and cross time zones or for those who must sleep during daytime hours. That's because their clocks are interrupted, which disrupts melatonin secretion, inevitably resulting in sleeplessness. Melatonin is often helpful for getting to sleep without the grogginess associated with tranquilizers.

Melatonin is also thought to keep us younger longer because of its antioxidant powers. A 1995 German study entitled "A Review of the Evidence Supporting Melatonin's Role as an Antioxidant" discussed in detail the reparative functions of melatonin on our bodies' cells. This revitalization is one of the fundamental steps in remaining younger looking and feeling.

Ongoing studies about melatonin suggest that it may also

- prevent and/or slow the growth of cancerous tumors
- aid in preventing Alzheimer's disease by inhibiting the process that causes amyloid plaques to spread through the brain, ultimately killing brain cells
- ease symptoms of premenstrual syndrome and menopause
- lessen the recurrence of cluster headaches
- lift depression related to seasonal affective disorder

Like the hormone DHEA, natural melatonin production decreases as we get older. Because of this, as well as its immune-enhancing qualities, some experts think melatonin may be an anti-aging substance.

A popular nutritional supplement, melatonin can be found in the form of pills, capsules, liquids, and sprays.

 ## RECOMMENDED USAGE

There is no RDI for melatonin.

Children
Administer only under the advice of a doctor or health practitioner.

Adults
300 micrograms daily.

CAUTION!

Melatonin is a hormone. As such, it should be used selectively and with care, because too much will inevitably affect your overall hormonal balance. It's not a supplement intended for pregnant or breastfeeding moms. Anyone suffering from autoimmune disease should also avoid melatonin, because it could hyperstimulate immune function. Furthermore, it may poorly react with prescription medications, especially tranquilizers. Take it only when you want to sleep, since it causes drowsiness.

METHIONINE
AND TAURINE

Overall Rating . . . . *Not Recommended to Supplement*

These two aminos are often grouped together because they contain sulfur and help manage the nervous system. Unlike cysteine, the third sulfuric amino, they don't help fight free radicals. Methionine's primary role is to help make taurine and cysteine. It also lowers the amount of histamine in our blood, a substance that in schizophrenics is often the culprit relaying garbled messages to the brain.

Taurine is needed to keep various nerves and muscles working smoothly and may also help maintain appropriate growth rate. Researchers are looking more closely at taurine because it may help treat illnesses such as epilepsy and cystic fibrosis.

 CAUTION!

Unless prescribed by a medical professional, it's not a good idea to take methionine or taurine supplements. In elevated amounts, both hamper the nervous system, potentially causing depression and short-term memory loss.

MILK THISTLE
(*Silybum marianum*)

Overall Rating. . . . . *Recommended*

For liver detoxification and support . . . . *Recommended*

If each of our organs were a person with a specific job, the liver would be the janitor. It's not a glamorous job because of all the cleaning, scrubbing, mopping, wiping, and backbreaking work involved.

Like a janitor, the liver cleans things up. It does its best to detoxify the nicotine in us after we smoke a cigarette, to scrub away the toxins from the environmental pollutants we breathe, to mop up the pesticides we eat from tainted foods, and to wipe down the mess we make of our bodies after a night of overindulging. Without a healthy, functioning liver, we don't do well. And sometimes our liver gets tired or dysfunctional because we ask it to work harder than it can.

Enter nature's doctor: milk thistle, a tall thorny plant with a bright maroon flower and seeds that look like a sunflower's. Surprisingly, this unassuming plant contains a combination of three flavanolignins known as silymarin, found in the fruit, seeds, and leaves of milk thistle. Together, these flavanolignins create the most potent liver protectors and rehabilitators known to humankind. German studies published in *Lehrbuch der Phytotherapie* as well as those in *Planta Medica* concur with overwhelming evidence that silymarin enhances and restores liver function because it acts as an antioxidant—with greater results than vitamin E—to fight off free radicals caused by alcohol and other liver toxins. And, unlike many pharmaceutical drugs, milk thistle has no side effects.

In Germany, milk thistle is used as the most prominent treatment for liver problems. With that in mind, consult with your physician about using it to effectively combat a variety of liver dysfunctions and other disorders, including

- cirrhosis
- chronic hepatitis A & B
- chemical poisoning
- mushroom poisoning
- fat intolerance
- gall bladder inflammation
- inflammation of bile ducts
- high blood pressure
- depression
- fatigue
- loss of appetite
- candida
- food allergies

Even people who don't drink or smoke are exposed to environmental toxins. If you experience chronic constipation, bloating, itchy eyes, menstrual difficulties, or emotional instability, your liver may not be functioning properly.

 ## RECOMMENDED USAGE

There is no RDI for milk thistle.

Milk thistle is available in tablets, which for best results should contain 20 to 35 milligrams of silymarin. To treat cirrhosis or hepatitis, take two to four capsules three times a day, after meals, for up to six weeks. Then reduce your intake to one capsule three times a day for up to six months.

You can also make a tea, tincture, or decoction from powdered seeds or other plant parts (preferably those parts that grow above ground). For tea, steep 1 teaspoon of seeds in boiling water for twenty minutes. Let the tea cool somewhat, but drink it while still hot.

Ten to forty drops of tincture or extract three times a day will help detoxify the liver, as will one cup of decoction three times a day for up to six months.

 CAUTION!

Liver problems are a serious matter, and you should always consult with a phyisician regarding treatment.

MOLYBDENUM

Overall Rating . . . . *Recommended*

For increasing energy . . . . *Not Recommended*

While the health conscious among us are busy reading labels to make sure we're getting enough folic acid; zinc; vitamins A, C, and E; and other supplements, it's nice to know that a few things we need tend to just take care of themselves. Molybdenum, a trace mineral, is one of these.

Trace minerals are just that: Minerals we need in our bodies but that do their job in amounts not exceeding a teaspoon. And although we don't need much and it's easy to get what we do need, these tiny amounts do mega-amounts of work.

Molybdenum, for example, is responsible for making an enzyme called xanthine oxidase, which enables our bodies to grow and develop properly. It's also known for

* helping our bodies utilize iron properly
* producing uric acid
* breaking down carbohydrates, fat, and protein so they can be used for energy

It's true that we don't need a lot of it, but just the same, a little bit of molybdenum is found within all our tissues. Exactly how much depends on where your food is grown. That's because we get molybdenum from the food we eat, and foods grown in mineral-rich soils provide us with more molybdenum than do foods that aren't. Given the decline of nutrient-rich soils on America's farms, it's not a bad idea to make sure your multivitamin contains molybdenum, which, fortunately, most of them do.

If you'd rather eat your daily dose of molybdenum from food than depend on it from a multivitamin, just munch good amounts of whole grains, eggs, dark green leafy vegetables, milk, lentils, sunflower seeds, macaroni, rice, noodles, and chicken, and you should be fine.

 ## RECOMMENDED USAGE

There is no such thing since there aren't any known deficiencies. There are, however, recommended amounts called "safe and adequate" amounts. They are as follows:

Children
15–250 micrograms

Adults
25–50 years: 75–250 micrograms
50+ years: 75–250 micrograms

As is typical for these numbers, they represent the least amount you need. So, if you're looking for amounts that may actually contribute to greater health (and so, happiness) rather than just stave off a deficiency, try between 50 and 500 micrograms per day.

 ## CAUTION!

Start yawning now, because there aren't any horror stories attached to molybdenum. Still, if you want to supplement, consult your doctor first if you have gout or high levels of uric acid.

MOTHERWORT
(*Leonurus cardiaca*)

Overall Rating . . . . *Recommended*

For alleviating PMS . . . . *Recommended*

For treating other gynecological conditions . . *Recommended*

To regulate menstrual cycle . . . . *Recommended*

It's unfortunate that the names of so many beneficial herbs are unattractive. Given what it does, motherwort might be better named mothercomfort or mothermaker. That's because this ancient herb can, among other things, calm the discomforts brought on by premenstrual syndrome (PMS) and regulate a sporadic period, thereby increasing the chances of getting pregnant for women who have had trouble.

The Latin name, *Leonurus cardiaca,* derives from the plant's appearance: It grows in tall spikes, with leaves jutting from the stem, resembling a lion's tail. Although motherwort is indigenous to Europe, it's been cultivated all over America.

Since Roman times, motherwort was known to help with a wide range of female problems. Today it is commonly used in combination formulas for both PMS and heavy periods, according to Janet Zand, O.M.D., and president of Zand Herbal. As mentioned, it can regulate periods (especially in conjunction with dong quai); it can promote labor and help relax the womb for a less stressful birth, as well as relieve postpartum pain; it also works well during menopause to cool those hot flashes and level out mood swings.

Motherwort is also believed to be an antispasmodic and good for blood, circulation, and the heart. To that end, you may want to consult with your doctor about using it to treat

* heart palpitations or a racing heart, especially in combination with hawthorn
* blood clots
* an overactive thyroid

Motherwort is also an effective overall relaxant, so you don't have to have problems with your period or your heart to benefit from its properties. And, by the way, it works well to promote urination.

 RECOMMENDED USAGE

There is no RDI for motherwort.

Children

Not advised for children. Administer only under the advice of a doctor or health practitioner.

Adults

You can find motherwort in most natural food stores in the form of tea, tincture, or capsules.

To treat most conditions listed above, drink three cups of the tea, or take 3 teaspoons of the tincture, per day. Or put forty drops of tincture in a cup of warm water and drink three times per day.

This herb doesn't work overnight. It may take several weeks for it to kick in. If you want to help stimulate labor, wait until approximately two weeks before your due date to drink the tea.

CAUTION!

Since motherwort is a uterine stimulant, avoid its use during pregnancy, or until your doctor determines it is time to induce labor. Also, if you have any kind of heart problem, work with a health care practitioner to determine the best course of action.

NIACIN
(Vitamin B₃)

Overall Rating.................. *Highly Recommended*

For promoting energy............ *Highly Recommended*

For lowering cholesterol.......... *Recommended*

It's kind of a contradiction. If you eat a big turkey dinner—as most of us do on Thanksgiving—the tryptophan in the turkey works with melatonin and seratonin to make you sleepy. At the same time, some of the tryptophan converts into niacin, which is one of the most important compounds for producing energy from foods. Maybe that's why some people doze off after that turkey dinner, while others go for a brisk walk.

Niacin, or vitamin B₃, is a member of that ever-critical B vitamin family that works in unison to keep us up and running. Niacin itself is known to

- release energy and provide antioxidant protection within cells
- team up with enzymes to convert carbohydrates into energy
- monitor the amount of glucose in blood
- lower cholesterol and blood triglyceride levels
- promote a healthy digestive system
- properly maintain the functions of estrogen, progesterone, testosterone, cortisone, and throxine
- maintain a healthy nervous system, skin, hair, and nails, especially with the assistance of riboflavin (vitamin B₂) and pyridoxine (vitamin B₆)
- help relieve symptoms of insulin-dependent diabetes mellitus

Perhaps the most exciting development regarding niacin is its impact on lowering cholesterol. In fact, American and European studies offered such favorable—and conclusive—results that *The Journal of the American Medical Association (JAMA)* recommended the use of niacin to reduce cholesterol.

When compared to cholesterol-lowering drugs, niacin supplements are far less expensive, have no side effects, and, from all sources, seem to reduce the number of heart attacks as well as heart disease–related deaths. All in all, niacin seems to work as well as some drugs.

Niacin supplements can also be used with drugs to successfully lower cholesterol. Either way, it's important to work with a doctor to tackle the cholesterol problem. *It can be detrimental to your health to suddenly start taking niacin if you're on cholesterol-lowering drugs, and even if you're not, a high dose of niacin is considered a drug and can be dangerous.* A doctor's supervision is, therefore, critical.

Niacin is also credited with widening blood vessels and improving circulation, which can reduce leg muscle cramps, dizziness or motion sickness, ringing in the ears, and vertigo associated with Ménière's disease. It may also prevent or treat migraine and PMS-related headaches, osteoarthritis, schizophrenia, and learning disabilities in children. And although some of those attributes are speculative, we know for a fact that niacin performs about fifty functions within our bodies that are essential for a healthy, active lifestyle.

Niacin is made up of two compounds: nicotinic acid and niacinamide. We get about half of our niacin from each. The nicotinic acid comes from food, while the amino acid tryptophan (remember the turkey?) converts into niacinamide within our bodies. To ensure this conversion, however, you must also have adequate amounts of biotin, thiamin, riboflavin, and pyridoxine. Remember—all the B vitamins work together to efficiently perform their jobs.

Although this may sound complicated, the good news is that it's easy to eat plenty of foods rich in either one of these compounds, ultimately providing us with all the niacin we need. Good sources include canned tuna, turkey breast, lamb, salmon, beef liver, chicken breast, pork roast, peanut butter, peanuts, rice, baked potatoes, peas, ground beef, asparagus, avocados, wheat germ, bagels, mushrooms, milk, flounder, cottage cheese, oatmeal, and any products "enriched" with niacin.

Unlike other B vitamins that are light or heat sensitive, niacin is hearty and can withstand most of the elements. Water is the exception, since it leeches out niacin. So if you cook your niacin-rich foods in water, just use a little bit.

 ## RECOMMENDED USAGE

Children
5–19 milligrams

Adults
25–50 years: 15–20 milligrams
50+ years: 13–15 milligrams

Since so many good foods are rich in niacin, deficiencies are very rare in developed countries. The exceptions include heavy alcohol drinkers and vegans, and especially vegan children, who eat little or no animal protein.

If you choose to supplement, whether to lower your cholesterol or because you don't eat from the animal protein menu, you may experience a flushed, red face and neck and an itching sensation as common side effects. These could last for as long as a day but are harmless. Be sure to take supplements on a full stomach, and drink some water, too, since it can help reduce the flush.

The amounts of niacin you need are determined by how much food you eat. Experts believe that we need 6.6 milligrams for every 1,000 calories consumed. A health-care professional can help with doses, but a typical supplement contains between 25 and 50 milligrams. If you take a nicotinic supplement, don't exceed 100 milligrams per day. Never take more than 2,000 milligrams per day of niacinamide supplements.

 CAUTION!

Up until the 1920s, niacin deficiencies were common, especially in poverty-stricken areas. The result was pellagra, a condition that includes dermatitis, diarrhea, memory loss, and confusion. If left untreated, pellagra is fatal.

In the 1920s, doctors realized that people on corn-rich but low-protein and low-dairy diets were most susceptible to pellagra. Once niacin-rich foods were introduced to those communities, the condition was reversed.

Of course, corn itself didn't cause the problem; rather, it's the hard skin around the kernel that makes it difficult to absorb niacin. Native Americans and Mexicans who prepared their corn with substances that loosened the skin didn't have pellagra.

People with high blood pressure, gout, diabetes, ulcers, and liver disease should consult a physician before supplementing.

Don't take niacin supplements with alcohol, sleeping pills, or estrogen.

PABA
(Para-aminobenzoic acid)

Overall Rating . . . . *Highly Recommended*

For sun protection (topically) . . . . *Highly Recommended*

To ease sun and other burns . . . . *Recommended*

For skin care . . . . *Recommended*

If you like to lounge around in the sunshine, you're probably aware of the good news about what para-aminobenzoic acid, or PABA, provides for your skin. Classic studies have proved its efficacy, and PABA is now a staple in most sun care products. In fact, it's an ingredient in most sunscreens because it blocks out the ultraviolet rays from the sun.

Although PABA isn't considered a vitamin, it is part of what makes up the folic acid molecule. Ironically, however, taking PABA supplements won't boost your levels of folic acid. In fact, taking it orally isn't recommended much at all. That's because our bodies make all the PABA we can use. If we ever do need a little extra, we can find it in foods like liver, kidney, molasses, sunflower seeds, eggs, yogurt, wheat germ, bran, brown rice, and other whole grains.

Considered an antioxidant for the skin, when applied topically PABA can also be used to

- treat vitiligo (discoloration of skin)
- ease the discomfort of burns
- maintain smooth, healthy skin

Two other important roles it plays is to help assimilate pantothenic acid and metabolize protein. Some unproven benefits include metabolizing amino acids and red blood cells; reversing gray hair to its original color; preventing hair loss; treating headaches, constipation, and anemia; relieving symptoms of arthritis; and preventing some wrinkles.

 ## RECOMMENDED USAGE

There are no known deficiencies, so no RDI has been assigned to PABA. If you want to see if it really does delay the arrival of wrinkles—or any other speculated benefit—consider simply taking a B-complex vitamin. There's typically plenty of PABA in those. But beware: If you're hoping to improve skin conditions, don't take oral supplements. Only creams and lotions containing PABA can do the trick.

 ## CAUTION!

Most health care professionals don't advise supplementing since we get all the PABA we need within our own bodies. Plus as little as 1 gram of a PABA supplement can cause nausea, vomiting, and diarrhea, rashes, and fever. Work with a doctor if you think you need to supplement.

PAU D'ARCO
(*Tabebuia species*)

Overall Rating . . . . *Not Recommended*

To combat symptoms of candida . . . . . . *Not Recommended*

For treating viral infections . . . . *Not Recommended*

For treating fungal infections . . . . *Not Recommended*

If you've ever suffered from candida, you probably know about pau d'arco. That's because it is one of the best remedies nature has to offer to combat the debilitating symptoms of candida, which include general fatigue, confusion, memory loss, depression, and recurrent yeast infections. In fact, candida is an overgrowth, and so an imbalance, of yeast within the body.

Pau d'arco, also known as taheebo or la pacho, is a large, deciduous, flowering tropical tree that grows in the Brazilian forests. It can reach heights of up to 100 feet and boasts a trunk with a circumference of 4 feet. The bark of this beautiful tree contains lapachol, the medicinal ingredient of pau d'arco.

Unknown to most of us, lapachol is an anticancer and antitumor agent, an organic antibiotic, and an effective treatment for candida.

It's also thought to be good for treating

- parasites
- fungal infections
- ringworm
- bronchitis
- colitis
- intestinal disorders
- thrush

Pau d'arco is widely available in the form of teas, tinctures, and capsules. Be mindful, however, that lapachol is the healing ingredient, which can only be acquired from mature trees. According to the *Journal of Herbs, Spices, and Medicinal Plants,* many pau d'arco products on the market these days are cultivated from trees with immature bark. The result? Little if any lapachol.

If possible, look for products that spell out that lapachol is contained in the product. Although that's about all you can do to ensure you're getting the good stuff, you can try working directly with an herbalist to get the highest quality product available.

 ## RECOMMENDED USAGE

There is no RDI for pau d'arco.

Children
Not advised for children. Administer only under the advice of a doctor or health practitioner.

Adults
To treat any of the conditions listed above, drink prepackaged tea on an empty stomach up to five times a day. If you can wrangle the raw bark from an herbalist, boil 15 to 20 grams of the bark in 1 pint of water. Let it boil and steep for fifteen minutes. Again, drink up to five cups a day on an empty stomach.

 ## CAUTION!

Watch out for tea made from immature bark.

PEONY
(*Paeonia officinalis*)

Overall Rating......................*Recommended*

For relieving menstrual discomfort and PMS . . *Recommended*
To regulate menstrual cycles............*Recommended*

Walk into a beautiful garden bursting with large flowers, and you might come upon the spectacular peony. This plant grows wild, as well as being a popular addition to many domestic gardens. It's a perennial plant that sprouts a large red or purplish red flower that seduces the eye with its glamour. But the part of this plant that we don't often see, the root, is as medicinal as the flower is lovely.

Traditionally used by the Chinese, the root of the peony can be made into tea or added to soups or wines to achieve its medicinal potential. Considered a tonic for the blood and circulation, it can be used to treat a variety of gynecological concerns, including PMS, menstrual cramps, irregular menstrual cycles, uterine bleeding, and anemia, says Daoshing Ni, O.M.D., of the Yo-San Institute of Chinese Medicine.

The peony's root is also thought to calm nervous anxiety, depression, and muscle spasms, while also being an effective pain reliever for skin conditions such as abscesses and boils.

 RECOMMENDED USAGE

There is no RDI for peony.

Children

Not advised for children. Administer only under the advice of a doctor or health practitioner.

Adults

If you'd like to try peony, go to the health food store and look only for the root. *The flower and stems are considered dangerous and should not be taken internally.*

Take the root and boil it in red wine. This herbal wine may even help with asthmatic problems.

You can also add the root to soup for good results, or drink it steeped in hot water as a tea.

 CAUTION!

Be very certain that you *only* drink concoctions from the root, *not* the flower, leaves, or stem, of this plant.

Avoid the herb if you are over fifty-five years of age. And don't give this herb to children. Drink it sparingly, and refrain from more than a few cups a day.

It's best to consult with a health care practitioner when using this herb. Doctors of Chinese medicine may be most knowledgeable with the medicinal purposes of peony.

PEPPERMINT
(*Mentha piperita*)

Overall Rating . . . . *Highly Recommended*

For treating gastrointestinal disorders . . *Recommended*

For easing headaches . . . . *Not Recommended*

For combating bad breath . . . . *Recommended*

Most of our diets probably include peppermint in the form of those red-and-white candies the waiter sometimes brings with our bill. The mints may seem like the perfect post-meal treat because they freshen our breath, but their purpose is actually twofold. That's because peppermint's primary use is to aid digestion. A hybrid of watermint and spearmint, peppermint is the most popular of all mints for therapeutic uses. These include relief from

- colon and stomach cramps, and nausea
- bloating, colic, and gas
- congestion and coughing
- overall aches and pains
- headaches and migraines

Peppermint is great at relieving gastrointestinal distress because it dispels gas, soothes the stomach, and gets bile flowing. Because it's an antispasmodic, it relieves all sorts of abdominal cramps, including those due to nausea, gas, and menstruation. Some women even drink peppermint tea and infusions for morning sickness. In other countries such as Britain and Denmark, peppermint is widely prescribed to treat irritable bowel syndrome.

Peppermint's essential oil contains menthol, which contributes to its ability to cool the skin, fight fungi and bacteria, break up respiratory congestion, and dull pain. And because it tastes so good, peppermint is used to flavor everything from confections and ice cream to toothpaste and lip gloss.

 ## RECOMMENDED USAGE

There is no RDI for peppermint.

This herb can be used by making an infusion from the leaves and tender stalks or by applying the essential oil. Peppermint is also available in capsule form.

The easiest way to reap the benefits of peppermint is to drink it in a tea or infusion. This method is used for digestive problems, headache, cough, and sore throat. The infusion may also be mixed with a lotion or ointment to relieve irritated skin. Peppermint massage and foot lotions are great for invigorating your muscles, as well as soothing hot, tired feet.

Peppermint's essential oil is very strong and an irritant. Therefore, it *must* be diluted in order to have a positive effect and should *only* be used externally. Diluted to 2 percent, it can be rubbed on the temples for headache pain. Mixing the oil into soaps, creams, and ointments produces means for antibacterial and antifungal cleansing, as well as pain relief. The diluted oil is also a good inhalant for respiratory congestion. In ointment form, it can complement this purpose when rubbed on the chest.

Peppermint capsules are most often used to treat irritable bowel syndrome.

CAUTION!

Because peppermint is an irritant, it must be used sparingly and, even then, only over short periods of time. Furthermore, it should *not* be given to children under the age of twelve. In some cases, peppermint has reduced lactation in breastfeeding mothers. Therefore, breastfeeding mothers should seek professional advice prior to using large amounts of this herb.

Finally, although the essential oil is popularly used to flavor a number of edible products, the oil itself should not be taken internally unless under professional supervision, as it may cause irritation.

PHENYLALANINE

Overall Rating . . . . *Recommended*

To improve mental abilities . . . . *Recommended*

You need adequate levels of phenylalanine to make the amino tyrosine because both work together to manufacture important brain chemicals such as dopamine, epinephrine, and norepinephrine. On its own, phenylalanine acts as a balm and invigorator for the mind because it is thought to

- lift depression
- increase memory retention
- heighten mental alertness

 RECOMMENDED USAGE

There is no RDI for phenylalanine.

Children
Administer only under the advice of a doctor or health practitioner.

Adults
Capsules
One 100-milligram capsule up to three times daily.

CAUTION!

Phenylalanine is not recommended if you're pregnant, have high blood pressure, suffer from skin cancer, or have the rare condition known as phenylketonuria (PKU). This includes avoiding the artificial sweetener, aspartame, which contains phenylalanine. When mixed with antidepressant medications, this amino acid may also give rise to dangerously high blood pressure.

Phenylalanine and tyrosine form tyramine, a substance that may induce migraine headaches. Those susceptible to migraine and vascular headaches should avoid phenylalanine and tyrosine supplements, as well as tyramine-filled foods, which include anything preserved, dried, or fermented, such as jams, pickles, cheese, raisins, and alcoholic beverages.

PHOSPHATIDYLSERINE (PS)

Overall Rating . . . . *Highly Recommended*

To increase memory capacity . . . . *Highly Recommended*

To stem memory loss . . . . *Highly Recommended*

For treating symptoms of Alzheimer's . . *Recommended*

"I'm sure we've met—what's your name again?"

"Give me a minute, it will come to me."

"I thought I put it right here."

Do you find yourself using these phrases more frequently or forgetting your keys or ATM password? We all have slips of memory from time to time, but for aging baby boomers trying to compete in the Information Age, memory has never been more critical.

That's why phosphatidylserine (or PS for short) is such welcome news to millions of aging Americans. PS, popular in Europe for years, has been found to be successful in helping the membranes of brain cells rejuvenate. With improved brain cell function—well, *voilà!*, increased memory capacity.

Dr. Thomas Crook, Ph.D., former chairman of both the National Institute of Mental Health and the American Psychological Association Task Forces on the Diagnoses and Treatment of Age-Associated Memory Impairment (AAMI), is a big fan of PS. In our book, *The Memory Cure*, we discuss the remarkable effects of PS on those suffering from AAMI and offer tips on boosting a failing memory.

Of course, this sounds too good to be true. But here's how it works: PS is already in our brain cells—in the internal layer of the cell membrane. There, it is actively involved in conducting information from one brain cell to another. In short, PS influences the neurotransmitters that help pass messages from one cell to another, much as a telephone operator helps relay messages from caller to receiver. By supplementing the aging cell membranes with a new infusion of PS, we can make sure that the messages continue to move quickly and effectively from one brain cell to the next. While our cells are being reinvigorated, so is our memory! To date, more than sixty studies have been published in medical journals, including *Aging* and *Neurology*, supporting the efficacy of PS to turn back the clock as much as twelve years for an aging brain.

We can naturally get PS in foods we eat, such as fish, rice, soy products, and those green leafy vegetables. In fact, it's hard not to get at least some PS every day. However, to work at therapeutic levels, we need to take a much higher dose that is readily available through our food.

In addition to memory improvement, PS can also

- enhance stress-coping mechanisms
- normalize brain biochemistry and physiology

Four separate studies in the last decade illustrate that PS can help with the symptoms of Alzheimer's disease (AD). The first two studies, from Italy, indicate that PS, taken at therapeutic levels, increases the cognitive functions of Alzheimer's patients and also improves their memory. Following these results, studies were conducted in the United States at Stanford and Vanderbilt Universities, with similar results.

There is consequently a theory that PS's ability to delay the memory deterioration component of aging may somehow be of use to researchers studying Alzheimer's disease. While this link has yet to be proven, it offers great possibilities for the future.

RECOMMENDED USAGE

There is no RDI for phosphatidylserine.

Children
Not recommended for children.

Adults
One 100-milligram tablet up to three times daily with meals.

 ## CAUTION!

Phosphatidylserine is not known to be toxic; however, memory loss may be a symptom of another illness or disorder. If you experience sudden confusion or memory loss, please consult your health-care practitioner.

PS is often sold as "PS complex," which includes other phospholipids and is only twenty percent PS, so look for 100-milligram tablets of pure PS to boost your memory.

Beware, however, of a similar product, phosphorylated serine, which is also available as a supplement but *does not work like PS and can cause adverse reactions.*

MEMORY

I find memory and how our brain works a fascinating topic. Together with Thomas Crook, Ph.D., a leading expert on aging and memory, I've written a book called *The Memory*

Cure. Several nutritional supplements, like gingko biloba, ginseng, and choline, have been touted as useful for enhancing memory and stemming the progression of memory loss that comes with normal aging. However, very little clinical research substantiates that these supplements are effective in improving memory. Gingko biloba, the most widely touted supplement, yields mixed results in studies. Some patients with dementia and Alzheimer's disease have improved, but there is no evidence gingko works for those with normal memory loss. The more definitive studies do show gingko to be an effective blood thinner, but that has nothing to do with memory.

In fact, only one supplement has been shown to have significant beneficial effects on improving memory. It is phosphatidylserine (PS). PS is a phospholipid that works in the brain to send chemical messages, as well as help the brain store and retrieve information. It has been shown clinically to enhance memory and improve your ability to concentrate.

Studies also show that PS will help maintain or even regain a high measure of cognitive brain function, including the ability to

- recognize faces
- remember easily forgotten details, such as names and telephone numbers
- recall accurately the content of conversations and professional discussions
- learn and remember new information
- maintain a high level of concentration
- improve verbal ability

On average, most people lose about 30 percent of their ability to memorize between the ages of fifty and seventy-five. That doesn't mean they forget what they already know, merely that they are that much less efficient in remembering new information. If you are concerned about a failing memory due to aging, PS is the nutritional supplement that really works.

PHOSPHOROUS

Overall Rating . . . . *Not Necessary to Supplement*

It turns out that phosphorous is the mineral behind the human. Rarely spoken of or celebrated, this hardworking substance contributes to some of our most significant processes. A sibling to calcium, phosphate is stored in our bones and teeth and keeps them strong. But where this mineral comes into its own is in our soft tissues, where it's also stored. Where, might you ask? Oh, just in every single one of our cells.

Phosphate is busiest while at work on our soft tissues because it helps create and manage energy; synthesizes protein, fat, and carbohydrates; fuses with fat to make phospholipids, which allow other substances to enter and exit cells; is a constituent of the nucleic acids, which are responsible for genetic information and cell replication; sends messages along our nerves; helps contract muscles, including the beating of our heart; stimulates hormone secretion; creates conditions that allow us to utilize B vitamins; and maintains the body's pH.

With all these amazing functions, you may wonder why this mineral is so overlooked. The reason is that phosphorus is just about in everything when it comes to mealtime, so we actually get too much without even trying. In fact, the trick lies more in curtailing our consumption of it than in augmenting our diets with more.

Every time you reach for a soda, you fill up on phosphorous. In addition to carbonated beverages, phosphorous is abundant in dairy products such as milk and cheese. This mineral is also found in beef, chicken, eggs, fish, and other types of red meat, as well as in most vegetables. Listing every source doesn't make sense, since there's a little bit of phosphorous in everything—even food preservatives.

 RECOMMENDED USAGE

Children
Not advised for children.

Adults
25+ years: 1,000 milligrams

Phosphate RDIs are not established for children, but like adults, children get more phosphate from their diets than they need. In fact, *supplementation for any age can be very dangerous.* No one should consider phosphate supplements unless suggested and supervised by a physician.

 CAUTION!

Phosphate deficiencies are rare. In fact, if you were deficient, you'd most likely be receiving medical care for serious illness such as kidney failure, starvation, or gastrointestinal disease. There are instances, however, when a very mild shortage may occur. Taking antacids that contain aluminum or magnesium for a long period of time can strip your body of phosphorous. Supplementation, even in this case, is very complicated and should be supervised by a medical professional.

Phosphorous is nontoxic, but high levels will deplete calcium, potentially leading to demineralization and osteoporosis. Be aware of phosphate intake, and be sure to take in twice as much calcium as phosphate, since these minerals should be balanced at a 1 to 2 ratio.

PSYLLIUM
(*Plantago ovata*)

Overall Rating. . . . . *Highly Recommended*

For effective elimination. . . . . *Highly Recommended*

For detoxification . . . . *Highly Recommended*

M any people might agree that a simple but workable philos-
ophy for life is to "go with the flow." Easier said than
done—especially when you're constipated and there is no flow to
go with.

Fortunately, nature provides us with psyllium, and when we mix
psyllium seeds with water and gulp them down, they expand—
eight to fourteen times their normal weight, in fact. The result?
Softened but bulkier bowels, which can move through us more
quickly and efficiently. In essence, after taking psyllium, we can
truly go with the flow!

But the advantages of taking psyllium go beyond relief from
constipation. Taking psyllium regularly is also thought to

- lower serum cholesterol levels
- reduce the desire to overeat
- assist diabetics since it reduces blood sugar
- ease the symptoms of irritable bowel syndrome
- reduce the possibility of varicose veins
- heal scraped internal tissues

In fact, psyllium is so effective for elimination and rejuvenation
that many doctors and practitioners are beginning to prescribe it

as a maintenance supplement for their patients, says Steven Bailey, N.D., professor at the Northwest Naturopathic College and author of the widely used detoxification protocol, *Passage 23*.

 RECOMMENDED USAGE

There is no RDI for psyllium.

Children

Not advised for children. Administer only under the advice of a doctor or health practitioner.

Adults

There are several ways to take psyllium. For treating constipation, you'll find it in over-the-counter products like Metamucil. More effective, however, is straight psyllium, without the other ingredients. You can find this at most health food stores in the form of wafers, capsules, seeds, and powder.

Add 1 teaspoon of the powder or seeds to a glass of water or juice, and drink immediately for good results. Whatever form you choose, however, it's best to drink two or three glasses of water when taking psyllium so it doesn't get clogged up midsystem.

If it's cholesterol you're targeting, studies show that taking psyllium twice a day can do the trick.

 CAUTION!

Avoid psyllium while pregnant or breastfeeding. And don't administer to children under age two.

People who have food allergies should consult a health care practitioner before supplementing with psyllium.

Don't take more than three doses per day. If you're taking too much, you'll experience gas, bloating, and diarrhea.

ROSEMARY
(*Rosemarinus officinalis L.*)

Overall Rating . . . . *Recommended*

For easing mood disorders . . . . *Recommended*

For improving circulation . . . . *Recommended*

To treat digestive disorders . . . . *Recommended*

For centuries, rosemary has been used to stimulate the nervous system, as well as the circulatory and digestive systems. Its analgesic, antiseptic, and anti-inflammatory properties may also make it useful for sprains, bruises, and eczema, as well as arthritis. In fact, rosemary is a common over-the-counter remedy in Great Britain where it's often used largely for its antiseptic and anti-inflammatory properties.

Among its many abilities, rosemary can also

- lift depression
- improve circulation
- stimulate digestion
- reduce colic and flatulence
- ease pain
- soothe skin conditions and abrasions.

In the brain, the neurotransmitter acetylcholine plays a signficant role in maintaining proper cerebral funtion. People who suffer from memory loss and Alzheimer's disease tend to have low levels of acetylcholine, which can be blocked by a substance called acetylcholinesterase. In addition to increasing blood circulation to the head, rosemary is thought to improve memory and ease depression because it prevents acetylcholinesterase from interfering with acetylcholine. This was studied in depth in both Germany and the Netherlands. Such an inhibiting effect protects the neurotransmitter and therefore helps maintain overall functioning of the brain.

On those days when your digestion seems to have "seized up," rosemary may provide some relief. It aids digestion by stimulating the gall bladder to release bile, while also reducing the buildup of intestinal gas, which causes flatulence, cramps, and colic.

Although more research is needed, rosemary might also prevent breast cancer. A 1996 study from Pennsylvania State University indicated that in lab rats, rosemary discouraged cancerous cells from attaching to healthy cells, which prevented the formation of tumors. While promising, one study is not a definitive finding.

 ## RECOMMENDED USAGE

There is no RDI for rosemary.

Children
Not advised for children. Administer only under the advice of a doctor or health practitioner.

Adults
This herb is available either fresh or dried, as an essential oil, and in capsule form.

Pour boiling water over the fresh or dried herb to make an infusion. You may drink the infusion to aid digestion and relieve indigestion. Added to an infusion that contains sage and lady's mantle, rosemary can be gargled to relieve a sore throat.

Add rosemary infusion or essential oil to shampoo to treat dandruff, or mix it with lotion to improve skin conditions and soothe aching muscles. Combined with an ointment, rosemary can help speed the healing of wounds. The infusion or essential oil may also be put into bath water to raise the spirits, treat wounds and aching muscles, and refresh the entire body.

A popular method to improve memory is to burn the essential oil (as in aromatherapy). Capsules may be taken to enhance memory, promote digestion, ease pain, and help prevent cancer.

 CAUTION!

In large doses, rosemary can be toxic. Furthermore, though rosemary may be used to stimulate the nervous and digestive systems, too much of it may result in overstimulation of these systems. This may lead to intoxication or agitation, which could worsen your symptoms. If you are considering using large amounts of rosemary, be sure to first consult a health care professional to ensure your well-being.

ROYAL JELLY

Overall Rating . . . . *Not Recommended*

To increase energy and sexual stamina . . . *Not Recommended*

For treating menopause . . . . *Not Recommended*

You have to admit, the queen bee has it pretty good. No, we're not talking about British royalty here, although there are similarities.

When bees are in the larva stage, they're fed the substance known as royal jelly, a milky fluid produced by the worker bees. But after the passing of three idyllic weeks, the royal jelly supply is cut off and reserved for the sole purpose of nourishing the queen. And nourish it does. The queen bee gets twice as big as the other female bees, has a much longer life span, and is about as fertile as fertile can be.

Royal jelly is packed with nutrients, including nearly all the important B vitamins and amino acids, and is full of minerals, including calcium, cobalt, iron, magnesium, potassium, phosphorous, and zinc. Aside from the many detectable substances in royal jelly, researchers believe there may be even more properties that make this jelly so special—properties they have yet to discover.

Aside from acting as a nutritional supplement, royal jelly is thought to work in conjunction with our hormones and our immune systems, because it may

- stimulate the adrenal glands
- increase energy

- help improve sex drive—mostly in men
- provide relief for problems related to menopause
- ease pain and stiffness due to arthritis
- act as a gentle antibiotic

However, none of these claims have been substantiated by research.

Some people use royal jelly to keep their skin looking young because they claim it minimizes wrinkles. Maybe so, maybe not, but research doesn't support this claim. Nontheless, many keep royal jelly in their medicine cabinet, hoping it might also relieve acne, reverse baldness, and lessen anxiety. Meanwhile, we'll keep watching the bees and pass on the "buzz" as soon as we learn something more.

You can get royal jelly in capsule form and break it open to apply directly to the skin.

 RECOMMENDED USAGE

There is no RDI for royal jelly.

Adults
Capsules
One 100-milligram capsule up to three times daily.

 CAUTION!

Royal jelly is not known to be toxic or have any adverse affects. Even though it's been around forever, we really know very little about royal jelly, and there is little research, so it should be taken in moderation. It's not recommended for women who are pregnant or nursing.

SAW PALMETTO

Overall Rating. . . . . *Recommended*

For treating benign prostate hypertrophy . . . . *Recommended*

The story goes that when some men reach middle age, they go through a bit of a crisis. So they buy a red sports car and some flashy new clothes, and maybe they'll even flirt with the idea of taking a young lover. But instead of claiming a new identity or finding romance, maybe what they really need is saw palmetto.

What does this little-known herb and middle-aged men have in common? The prostate gland. In fact, both studies and anecdotal evidence have made saw palmetto one of the most widely sought-after supplements on the market today!

Around their fortieth year, men experience hormonal changes so that by the time they're fifty, they are susceptible to a condition known as benign prostate hypertrophy (BPH). That's when dihydrotestosterone compels the cells in the prostate gland to multiply excessively, thus enlarging the prostate gland. When that happens, some rather unpleasant things result, such as frequent urination during the night, difficulty urinating, and an interrupted flow—or dribbling—during urination.

There are drugs for an enlarged prostate, but one of the possible side effects is—uh-oh—a loss of libido! The moral of the story? No fancy red sports car on earth will motor up a man if drugs are keeping him down.

Saw palmetto, on the other hand, contains something called liposterolic extract, which inhibits the dihydrotestosterone. What that means, ultimately, is if you have an enlarged prostate, saw palmetto may help control it. So, if you're over forty, go to the health food store before you head for the car lot. You'll be better off no matter what you drive.

As an added benefit, your sex drive might be better, too. Saw palmetto is also known as an aphrodisiac for men. Who would think that a scrubby little palm tree found mostly in Florida and the West Indies would produce a berry with such virile effects!

For men who have cystitis or an inflamed urinary tract, saw palmetto can help those conditions as well.

This herb is available as decoctions, tinctures, or tablets.

 ## RECOMMENDED USAGE

There is no RDI for saw palmetto.

Children
Not advised for children. Administer only under the advice of a doctor or health practitioner.

Adults
The amount of saw palmetto you take will be determined by the form in which you take it. A health care practitioner can assist you here. It's safe to say, however, that in tablet form, you can take up to 500 milligrams three times a day. Be sure that whatever supplement you use contains 85 percent fatty acids and sterols (liposterolic extract).

CAUTION!

There are no known toxic reactions to saw palmetto.

If you believe you have an enlarged prostate, be sure to have a complete medical exam, including a prostate-specific antigen (PSA) test, and consult with your doctor about using this herb.

SELENIUM

Overall Rating . . . . *Highly Recommended*

To prevent against free
radical damage. . . . . *Highly Recommended*

For producing the thyroid hormone . . . *Highly Recommended*

To prevent heart attacks. . . . . *Highly Recommended*

To prevent prostate cancer . . . . *Highly Recommended*

Ever notice how kids love to get dirty? They play in dirt, they relish in it—sometimes they even eat it. Perhaps that's because they instinctively know that the cool clumps of earth that so often collect under their fingernails and behind their ears are vital for life as we know it. The foods we eat absorb many of their nutrients from the soil in which they're grown. One such nutrient is selenium, a trace mineral that is concentrated in soil and may help our bodies fight all kinds of ailments.

Experts have gone back and forth about whether or not selenium is good for us. It was originally thought to be essential for animals but harmful for people. In fact, only recently has science begun to consider the powerful benefits that selenium may offer.

Perhaps most important, selenium is an essential ingredient of glutathione peroxidase, a potent antioxidant made in our bodies, which defends us against free radicals. For this purpose, selenium works best with vitamins A and E. These three substances enhance one another's performance, combining their abilities and taking them to a higher level. With that in mind, consider that adequate levels of selenium are thought to help

- fight breast, colon, lung, and prostate cancer
- prevent hardening of the arteries, strokes, and heart attacks
- lift depression and increase mental acuity in the elderly
- relieve arthritis, acne, and dermatitis, when used in conjunction with vitamin E
- remedy the toxic effects of arsenic, copper, and mercury
- mobilize the thyroid hormone

If the golden years are approaching, be sure to keep a good supply of selenium on hand. Age-old studies have shown that it can reduce age-related illness by inhibiting virtually all the mechanisms that lead to physical and mental deterioration. A newer German study, reported in *Ernahrungswiss,* supports this by concluding that the antioxidant functions that stimulate the thyroid also maintain other metabolic functions. Some nutritionists think that with more studies, it may become the number one anti-aging remedy. So how do we get enough selenium?

American farmlands have been stripped of selenium, leaving our foods deficient of this essential mineral. Animal products that contain selenium include organ meats, beef, chicken, and seafood—but only if the animals were fed selenium-rich nutrients. The same is true of plant foods: If broccoli, garlic, onions, red grapes, oatmeal, brown rice, and other whole grains were raised in selenium-rich soil, these foods will retain concentrations of it. But it's just about impossible to know the nature of the soils in which our foods are grown.

The only alternative is supplementing. And here's another good reason to supplement: Cooking foods robs them of selenium. So does processing them. Supplementation is clearly the only way to know you're getting enough.

Selenium is widely available in supplemental forms. It's best to go with either "yeast-based" or "organic" types. Other nonorganic formulas, such as selenate and sodium selenate, tend to be difficult to absorb and may be a waste of money. You may also find selenium as part of a good multivitamin supplement.

 ## RECOMMENDED USAGE

RDIs have not been established for selenium, but experts differ on suggested intake. Some encourage from 100 micrograms to 200 micrograms per day for adults, while others recommend up to 400 micrograms per day for adults who live in areas with selenium-poor soil. Your safest bet is to stick to 100 micrograms per day.

 ## CAUTION!

Most of us tend to be low in selenium due to soil depletion. People who are exposed to toxic chemicals, smokers, the elderly, and vegetarians have the highest risk of deficiencies, resulting in sore or weak muscles.

Supplementing with more than 2,400 micrograms a day can be toxic. This will manifest as the odoriferous and unmistakable stink of garlic in your breath, sweat, and urine. If this happens, discontinue use and call your physician.

Selenium has been linked to birth defects and therefore should be avoided by pregnant women or women trying to conceive.

SHARK CARTILAGE

Overall Rating . . . . *Recommended*

For reducing cancerous tumors . . . . *Recommended*

For relieving arthritis. . . . . *Not Recommended*

They're scary. They have sharp teeth. They're ugly. And they've been known to kill people, or at least munch on people's body parts. We don't plan our summer vacations around going to Florida and swimming with them. They've been portrayed as sea monsters in movies. And certain professionals with questionable ethics have been nicknamed after them. So it's clearly a switch to think of sharks as lifesavers, but, when all is said and done, that may in fact be what they can offer humankind.

Very little research has been done to prove pulverized shark cartilage can decrease malignant tumors in cancer patients. But enough has been demonstrated, in particular by Dr. I. William Lane, to warrant further study. And so, recently the Food and Drug Administration (FDA) agreed to fund studies that will tell us more about what Dr. Lane swears by. He began his studies after dwelling on the well-established fact that, while other sea animals get sick, sharks are virtually disease-free. That includes cancer. Then, in 1983, two researchers from the Massachusetts Institute of Technology (MIT) reported that shark cartilage contains something that prevents the development of blood vessels that nourish tumors, so the tumors can't grow. Studies from Harvard University backed up the notion, stating that if you can inhibit angiogenesis, or the development of new blood networks, you can prevent the growth of cancer-ridden tumors.

In self-funded studies, Dr. Lane traveled the globe to work with cancer patients for whom conventional treatment—radiation therapy and chemotherapy—had not worked. He utilized cartilage from the fin of the shark—which is made up of protein, ash, water, calcium, phosphorous, amino acids, carbohydrates, and mucopolysaccharides (that's what apparently inhibits the tumor growth)—and gave it to these patients, either rectally or orally. In the follow-up studies he was able to conduct (finances weren't always available, so not all studies could be tracked) Dr. Lane discovered significant results. Although the procedure didn't help everyone, several patients went on to live for years longer, while still others eventually showed absolutely no sign of cancer, were able to resume normal lives and activities, and are still alive today. All the patients in Dr. Lane's most famous study were considered fatally ill when they began the trial.

But treating cancerous tumors is just the biggest news about what shark cartilage might be able to do. Because of its anti-inflammatory properties, as well as its other nutrients, some believe it may also be good for treating broken bones, osteoporosis, and arthritis. However, no studies confirm these uses, although shark cartilage is widely touted to ease the symptoms of arthritis.

There have been no side effects with the use of shark cartilage in the studies conducted so far.

 ## RECOMMENDED USAGE

There is no RDI for shark cartilage.

Shark cartilage is available in bulk powder form, which can be mixed with water or juice and drunk. It can also be mixed with water and taken as an enema, which is often the most effective means for cancer patients in advanced stages.

You can also buy shark cartilage in gelatin capsules or caplets. This can be hard on your stomach, however, since you must take it in such high doses.

Finding purely processed shark cartilage may prove difficult, since there are no standards and since there may be manufacturers motivated more by greed than by promoting the health and well-being of their customers. Because this is a new product on the American market, you might want to research how to locate the purest form of it. Books are available about both the product and how best to use it. There's also a great deal of information on the Internet, but beware of manufacturers simply trying to sell more of their products.

 ## CAUTION!

Since there is no conclusive evidence that taking shark cartilage will successfully reduce tumors or treat cancer, you will be using it at your own risk. Most people agree that it's best used by cancer patients who have had little or no luck with conventional methods of treatment. Consult with your physician before starting supplementation to make sure it won't interfere with existing treatment.

Pregnant women, children, or people who have just undergone surgery should absolutely *not* use shark cartilage.

SLIPPERY ELM
(*Ulmus fulva*)

Overall Rating . . . . *Recommended*

For relieving cough . . . . *Recommended*

For alleviating gastrointestinal
distress . . . . *Recommended*

D o you remember climbing trees as a kid? The feeling of being on top of the world with the greatest of bird's-eye views? The sound of the leaves and the intimacy with tree creatures? It was both an exhilarating and soothing experience. Chances are good, if you grew up in the United States, one of the trees you climbed was an elm.

Even though your tree climbing days may be over (then again, maybe not!), you can still enjoy a pleasant relationship with these great deciduous trees. Only now, you can reap the soothing benefits of the elm's bark.

Slippery elm, as it's called, is one of the best herbs going to soothe inflamed or sensitive mucous membranes. In fact, it has such a long-standing reputation that many over-the-counter cough relief preparations are formulated with slippery elm.

Taken as a tea, it's thought to be an excellent remedy for all types of gastrointestinal disorders, including ulcers, nausea, indigestion, colitis, diarrhea, food allergies, and heartburn, and is used in medical institutions worldwide.

This common herb not only helps us heal on the inside, it works on the outside, too. By mixing slippery elm powder with water, you'll have a good poultice for wounds or skin conditions such as eczema, gangrene, bedsores, burns, boils, tumors, or diaper rash. It might also draw out stubborn splinters.

The herb may also be useful for anyone recovering from a severe illness. Drinking it as a tea or eating porridge made from the powder has effectively helped babies, the elderly, and everyone in-between recovering from illness, with soothing, nutritional results.

In lozenge form, it can also ease nausea caused by pregnancy or motion sickness. Some even believe it can curb the desire for nicotine.

 ## RECOMMENDED USAGE

There is no RDI for slippery elm.

To make a tea decoction, mix one part powdered bark to eight parts water. Boil and simmer for fifteen minutes. Drink one cup three times a day for stomach upset or throat irritations.

This herb is available as a decoction, in powder form, or in tablets. Follow the directions as printed on the label.

 ## CAUTION!

There are no toxic reactions to slippery elm. If, however, you have a reaction, consult a health care practitioner.

SOY

Overall Rating . . . . *Highly Recommended*

As a source of complete protein . . . . . *Highly Recommended*
For treating osteoporosis . . . . *Highly Recommended*
To alleviate symptoms of menopause . . *Highly Recommended*

Some words of advice: If you ever find yourself stranded in a northern Chinese desert—go for the soybeans! At least that's what's suggested by the legend surrounding the discovery of the soybean: In 1500 B.C., two warlords eluded starvation by eating what are now thought to be the early soybean's ancestor. Of course, even if we never get near a Chinese desert, most of us might want to consider getting closer to soy. Although the uses for soy are varied, ultimate survival is still on the list. That's because in addition to being highly nutritious, vegetarian, and low-fat, soy is also thought to

- protect the heart by lowering cholesterol and triglycerides and by reducing blood pressure
- offset the symptoms of menopause, including hot flashes, vaginal dryness, and irritability
- aid in digestion

Soy is making news because it is a complete protein, which means it contains all eight of the essential amino acids. Even better, it has more protein per gram than eggs, meat, fish, or cheese—and it's lower in saturated fat and calories. Soy also contains other nutrition biggies, such as the B vitamins, bioflavonoids, calcium, vitamin E, lecithin, magnesium, and omega-3 fatty acids. Soybeans are also very high in fiber, which aids in digestion and keeps the colon healthy.

In addition to its nutritious composition, soy contains a number of nonnutritive substances that fight cancer. The most important of these are phytic acid, protease inhibitors, and isoflavones. Phytic acid is an antioxidant known to arrest tumor growth in lab animals. Protease inhibitors block enzymes that cause cancer. Furthermore, cells that have been exposed to cancer or have become cancerous may revert to their original healthy state after being exposed to protease inhibitors.

Isoflavones are compounds similar to human estrogen, which is thought to play a role in breast cancer. Isoflavones compete with estrogen in the body and may prevent the hormone, which is stronger, from binding with cells and causing damage. Two isoflavones, genistein and daidzien, are considered most important for fighting breast cancer. Genistein has a special ability because it appears to prevent tumors (of varying cancers, including prostate), from developing the blood vessels they need to grow. Nonetheless, no studies have confirmed soy's direct benefits regarding cancer.

Because isoflavones are so similar to estrogen, they may help women undergoing menopause by relieving a number of the discomforting symptoms that occur when the body ceases to produce its own estrogen. For some women, they may be a good alternative to estrogen replacement therapy, which may increase the risk of developing certain cancers such as breast cancer. There are few things most researchers agree on, but here's one: Eat soy!

It's well known that consuming fewer high-calorie/high-fat foods is one way to help reduce high blood pressure, clogged arteries, and high cholesterol. Soy foods lend themselves to this function by being naturally low-cal and low-fat, but they have also been shown to reduce "bad," or LDL, cholesterol and triglycerides, as well as raise "good," or HDL, cholesterol. While how it does so has yet to be determined, soy may help reduce heart disease and strokes by relieving these cholesterol-related conditions.

 ## RECOMMENDED USAGE

There are no RDIs for soy, but, for maximum benefit, experts recommend getting from 20 to 50 grams of soy each day. The best way to reap the benefits of soy is to add it to your diet.

The most popular soy foods are tofu and soy milk. Tofu is a bean curd that comes in various textures. Firm and soft tofu can be cooked and are good in soups, stews, stir-frys, and pasta dishes. Silken tofu, which is creamier, is best blended and mixed into recipes such as creamy soups, sauces, dips, baked goods, and drinks. Soy milk is a worthy alternative to regular milk. It's lactose-free, comes in varying flavors, and can be imbibed hot or cold. Also well known is soy sauce, which contains soy protein. Its high salt factor, however, may not be good for people with high blood pressure or heart disease.

For most of us, a less-familiar soy food is tempeh, a chewy, fermented soybean patty that's a great substitute for meat because it can be fried, grilled, or chopped. If ground beef is what you're craving, a product called textured soy protein might do the trick. When mixed with hot water, textured soy protein can be used in chili, spaghetti sauce, sloppy joes, and burgers—any recipe that calls for ground beef.

Two other sources of soy are soy flour and soy isolates. Soy flour, the base ingredient for textured soy protein, can be mixed into any recipe that calls for flour. Soy isolates are nutritional supplements that are high in cancer-fighting substances such as isoflavones, protease inhibitors, and phytic acid. A number of soy powders are on the market and can be mixed into juices or shakes. When purchasing these powders, be sure that soy isolates are listed first or second in the ingredients. That's because some powders are made of soy flour, which isn't as high in isoflavones, protease inhibitors, and phytic acid.

Of course, our grocery stores are filled with various soy lunch meats, soy hot dogs, soy ice creams, and the like. But don't rely on these as the best source of soy proteins and isolates. Like other highly processed foods, much of the nutritional content is compromised by the time it gets to you.

 CAUTION!

Soy is not known to have any toxic effects. Some soy products, however, such as soy sauce, miso, and natto, are fermented and contain high levels of salt. *These products could dangerously elevate the blood pressure of people on certain antidepressant medications.* If you take antidepressants, be sure to consult with your health practitioner prior to consuming high amounts of these soy foods.

ST. JOHN'S WORT
(*Hypericum perforatum*)

Overall Rating. . . . . *Recommended*

For combating depression. . . . . *Highly Recommended*

For treating bipolar disorder. . . . . . . *Not Recommended*

L ife demands a lot of us. We have to work. We have to work out. We have to grocery shop, houseclean, and keep up with household repairs. Some of us are raising kids, and that's a very big job. Then there's turning on the news and being confronted with curing the ills of the world: cleaning up pollution, overcoming violence, saving endangered species, and feeding hungry children in third-world countries—or right here in the United States.

It's enough to bring on the blues.

Depression has reached staggering new heights in America. It's likely that everyone knows someone on Prozac, Xanax, Zoloft, or St. John's wort. That's right, St. John's wort, a wild, perennial shrub that grows all around the world and has been the choice treatment for depression in Germany for years. Finally, in America, it's competing neck-in-neck with the expensive prescription drugs that can impose pages and pages worth of side effects on the user.

Back in the 1970s, the Soviet medical journal *Vrachebnoe Delo* heralded St. John's wort as an effective treatment for physiological problems associated with the brain. In the 1980s, the *British Medical Journal* reported that the herb was as effective as any antidepressant prescription drug. And at last, in 1997, a book published in America entitled *Hypericum and Depression,* by

Harold Bloomfield, confirmed that, without serious side effects, St. John's wort works well to treat mild depression.

People who take the herb for this purpose say it's a subtle, but effective, mood elevator. Be prepared for the herb to take four to six weeks to do what it does so well. But given that it's inexpensive, available in health food stores and grocery stores alike, and has only one (avoidable) side effect after prolonged use, most people think it's worth the wait.

With all the attention St. John's wort has gotten of late for treating depression, you might think that's all it's good for. Not so. It's been among the most commonly used herbs for centuries to help

- heal wounds
- relieve discomfort associated with eczema, psoriasis, shingles, cold sores, herpes, hemorrhoids, vaginal infections, mild burns, and sunburns
- ease back pain caused by sciatica and rheumatism
- calm emotional disturbances related to menopause and neuralgia or general irritability
- attack viral infections, from the flu to HIV
- expedite healing and treat pain from postpartum trauma to perineum or coccyx
- soothe digestive problems
- prevent tetanus
- alleviate incontinence

Although unproven, a poultice made up of several herbs, but primarily St. John's wort, might even treat basal cell carcinoma, a form of skin cancer. It could also depress the appetite if taken with ephedra.

Given that it is all it's cracked up to be, you may want to keep some St. John's wort in your medicine cabinet. It's available as a tea, tincture, oil, poultice, wash, salve, and in capsules.

RECOMMENDED USAGE

There is no RDI for St. John's wort.

Children
Not generally advised for children, though it may be used as an alternative to Ritalin, a common prescription drug for children with attention deficit disorder. Administer only under the advice of a doctor or health practitioner.

Adults
To treat depression, take two 300-milligram capsules up to three times daily. It can be taken all at once or spread throughout the day. Remember—it may take a while for St. John's wort to work, but it's worth it.

Consult a health care practitioner or reference books for specific remedies to other conditions.

 ## CAUTION!

Some fair-skinned people may find that after taking St. John's wort for a prolonged period of time, they become sensitive to the sun or may break out in rashes when exposed to the sun. To prevent this, always use sunblock—which you should in any case. If that doesn't help, consult a health care professional.

TEA
(*Camellia sinensis*)

Overall Rating. . . . . *Recommended*

To boost the immune system . . . . *Recommended*

From the precise brewing ceremonies practiced by Japanese geishas to the customary practice of taking afternoon tea in Great Britain to curling up on the couch with a mug and a good book, no other beverage has as many cultural and historical rituals associated with it as tea.

Although there is a wide variety of teas—each imparting their own flavor and preferred at different times of the day and in different parts of the world—basic tea comes in only three varieties: green, oolong, and black. All three types are made from the leaves of the same plant, but they differ in how the leaves are dried and the degree to which they are allowed to ferment. Green tea is not fermented, oolong tea is partially fermented, and black tea is fully fermented.

Regardless of fermentation, tea is a stimulant and an astringent. That means it's good for when you have a cold since it helps dry and clear fluids (such as phlegm) from your body. And by toning the intestinal tissues, it also works well as a digestive aid. Plus, it's a great source of potassium, magnesium, and folic acid (vitamin B_9, the vitamin that helps protect against spinal birth defects). So the Japanese ritual of drinking a cup of green tea after nearly every meal isn't a bad idea. And it's backed up by decades of impressive research from the East.

Given that green tea is also thought to boost the immune system, perhaps the Western world should put the kettle on: Polyphenols, which are found in tea, may act as antioxidants, which eliminate harmful substances and help cells withstand damage and remain healthy. Polyphenols may also benefit the circulatory system by preventing the buildup of cholesterol and strengthening blood vessels. Green tea also contains catechins, which are thought to ward off viral infection and protect against cancers of the colon, stomach, and skin.

If you're feeling immortal and don't concern yourself with such things, here's something to smile about: Green tea is full of fluoride and may help prevent cavities. And you can place a damp tea bag, or poultice made from damp, loose tea leaves, to relieve itching and swelling from an insect bite.

Like green tea, oolong may strengthen blood vessels, limit cholesterol absorption, and reduce the risk of atherosclerosis, or hardening of the arteries.

Black tea is fully fermented and rich in tannins or tannic acid, a natural antiseptic. You can relieve some discomfort caused by minor cuts and bruises by applying a fresh, cool tea bag to them. Drinking a strong cup of cold black tea can combat diarrhea, while weak cold black tea can be washed over a sunburn for some short-term relief. A steaming cup of tea with lemon and honey is a traditional folk remedy for hoarseness. And if you get headaches and don't mind the effects of caffeine, a strong cup of hot tea can provide some relief. Tired eyes? Try lying down and placing a cool, damp tea bag on each eye. If nothing else, your body will probably appreciate the rest.

 ## RECOMMENDED USAGE

There is no RDI for tea.

Children

Administer only under the advice of a doctor or health practitioner.

Adults

Capsules
One 100-milligram capsule up to three times daily.
Tea
Three cups green tea daily, or 300–400 milligrams once daily.

 CAUTION!

Tea contains caffeine and other natural stimulants. While these stimulants may have a positive effect on the body, they can also have a negative effect if an excessive amount is consumed. Dietary caffeine has been linked to conditions such as insomnia, indigestion, and fibrocystic breast disease. A good rule of thumb is to limit your intake of tea to two cups per day, unless your health care practitioner directs you differently. Those with stomach problems may want to avoid drinking tea completely, since it can stimulate the production of acid. If you are being treated for asthma, you may want to consult a doctor before drinking tea on a regular basis.

TRYPTOPHAN

Ever notice how tired you feel after a big turkey dinner? Much of your drowsiness may have been the cause of tryptophan, the amino acid that is abundant in turkey. Tryptophan plays a major role helping us sleep and relax. This "mellow" amino is thought to

* relieve insomnia
* soothe anxiety
* lessen the effects of jet lag
* ease migraines

 CAUTION!

In 1989, tryptophan supplements were recalled by the FDA because they caused flulike side effects. Therefore, supplements are not recommended. It is harmless, however, to increase your intake of tryptophan through natural food sources such as avocados, bananas, cheese, peanuts, and turkey.

TYROSINE

Overall Rating . . . . *Not Recommended*

For Depression . . . . *Recommended*

A s mentioned previously, we need tyrosine and phenylalanine to create the brain chemicals that regulate our moods, sleep cycles, and other biochemical processes. On its own, this amino acid is thought to

- lift depression
- reduce anxiety and stress
- energize the mind
- curtail the irritability and depression associated with PMS

Tyrosine has also been used to help cocaine addicts kick their habit. They claim that the amino mitigates some of the worst symptoms of cocaine withdrawal, including depression, exhaustion, and temperamental behavior. However, no scientific evidence has confirmed this.

 RECOMMENDED USAGE

There is no RDI for tyrosine.

Children
Administer only under the advice of a doctor or health practitioner.

Adults

Capsules

One 100-milligram capsule up to three times daily.

 CAUTION!

Tyrosine and phenylalanine also form tyramine, a substance that may induce migraine headaches. Those susceptible to migraine and vascular headaches should avoid phenylalanine and tyrosine supplements, as well as tyramine-filled foods, which include anything preserved, dried, or fermented, such as jams, pickles, cheese, raisins, and alcoholic beverages.

Tyrosine may also dangerously elevate the blood pressure if combined with some antidepressant medications. If you take such medications, be sure to consult with a physician before using tyrosine supplements.

VALERIAN
(*Valeriana officinalis*)

Overall Rating . . . . *Recommended*

For relaxation . . . . *Recommended*

To sleep better . . . . *Recommended*

Let's say it's Mother's Day and you're running late for the celebration. You forgot to get a present and feel embarrassed, but rather than be any later, you keep driving, feeling guilty.

Then, a miracle: You spy a beautiful crop of wildflowers growing along the side of the road. The stems are tall and erect, the tiny flowers a pretty pink or white—surely nice enough for a Mother's Day bouquet. You stop the car, dash out with your pocketknife, ready to cut them for your bouquet when—whoa! The odor just about knocks you off your feet. In fact, they smell like feet! Sorry, Mom—no gift this year.

In this scenario, there's both good and bad news about having come upon the valerian plant. Although the Greek physician Galen called this plant *phu* for its malodor, (which means it's not going to the party), it is renowned for having a calming effect. So as you drive away from the flowers, you might actually feel a little more relaxed about not bringing Mom a gift.

The medicinal properties of the valerian plant are housed in its root. The plant's calming effect, which works well for insomnia, is from valepotriates, a substance that actually depresses the central nervous system. Several studies published in *Planta Medica* back this up: They claim that taking valerian before going to bed can reduce the time it takes you to fall asleep while also improving the quality of your sleep. For most people, it works as well or better than over-the-counter or prescription sleep aids because, though it knocks you out at night, the effects wear off by the time you need to wake up. So no irritating grogginess to battle with when the sun rises.

Not everyone has perfect luck with valerian, however. Some people, about 5 percent, experience the opposite affect. It's wise, therefore, to start with low doses. Store-bought capsules will provide doses on the label. Go for one capsule to start with, so you'll know if it works for you. If it doesn't, you might try a different brand. Sometimes, for mysterious reasons, that works.

Valerian is a component in more than 100 drugs in Germany, where it is considered a safe and effective soothing agent. You won't find valerian as the main ingredient in drugs in the United States, however. That's because you can't get a patent on plants, and drug companies will only study and utilize what they can patent.

In addition to its soporific qualities, valerian is thought to be effective in treating

- epilepsy
- high blood pressure
- stress or anxiety
- tension headaches
- muscles spasms or rheumatism
- stomach upset or indigestion

Cats love the smell of valerian, so if you plant a bed of it outside, your feline friend will be forever grateful. But beware: Rats also like the smell, so be sure you have the cat to chase them off so you're not surprised by unwanted pests.

RECOMMENDED USAGE

There is no RDI for valerian.

Children
Not advised for children. Administer only under the advice of a doctor or health practitioner.

Adults
Capsules
Two 400-milligram capsules up to four times daily.
Tincture
Three drops in an 8-ounce glass of water three times daily.

You can purchase valerian in capsules or make a tea, tincture, or poultice.

To treat rheumatism or sore muscles, make a poultice by diluting and heating a tincture, pour it on a cloth, and place the cloth directly on the sore area.

You can make tea with ten to sixteen drops of tincture in water, but be warned—it doesn't taste good. Or take 1 teaspoon of ground root in 1 pint of water. This is best when cold.

For a soothing bath, add tincture drops to bath water.

Consult with a health care practitioner for specific doses to treat other conditions.

 CAUTION!

Don't use for more than three weeks without taking a break or you risk depression. Overdosing causes vomiting, as well as depression.

VITAMIN A
(Beta-carotene)

Overall Rating . . . . *Highly Recommended*

For cell growth . . . . *Highly Recommended*

For reproductive functioning . . . . *Highly Recommended*

For strong bones . . . . *Recommended*

To support the immune system . . . . . . *Highly Recommended*

To treat glaucoma . . . . *Not Recommended*

For reducing stress . . . . *Recommended*

To process free radicals . . . . *Recommended*

When you take those long road trips from one end of the country to the other, you can thank vitamin A for your ability to drive through the night. Good vision, especially at night, is the result of vitamin A enabling proper function of the retina.

In fact, vitamin A, in concert with critical enzymes, promotes healthy cellular growth throughout our bodies. It also is thought to

- discourage infections of the respiratory and intestinal tracts
- enrich and support the overall immune system
- repair damaged DNA
- promote healthy bones, teeth, skin, and hair
- maintain healthy mucus membranes
- expedite healing of rheumatic fever and infectious hepatitis.

Although the results from studies are still being evaluated, some experts believe vitamin A can also treat glaucoma. Others believe that it can ease physical conditions resulting from air pollution and alleviate stress, says Dr. Leon Chaitow of London, England. "Vitamin A is a great balancer of the body's systems," he says, "which is why it is essential to get an adequate amount."

Even though we are highly dependent on vitamin A, neither plants nor animals actually contain it. Rather, plants comprise water-soluble beta-carotene, which our bodies convert into vitamin A. Animal products consist of a fat-soluble precursor to vitamin A, called preformed or provitamin A. Once ingested, our bodies produce a chemical change to turn the precursors into vitamin A.

Beta-carotene is the preferred source of vitamin A since it is both water soluble and an antioxidant. That means by eating apricots, asparagus, broccoli, cantaloupes, carrots, spinach, cabbage, kale, mustard greens, red peppers, squash, sweet potatoes, peas, and oranges, you will fight off those pesky free radicals, contributing to cellular demise, which often results in cancer and heart disease, as concluded by studies in the United States, England, and elsewhere.

Among the animal products that provide the fat-soluble version of the vitamin are beef, chicken and fish liver, salmon, swordfish, sole, butter, cheese, and eggs. But if you need to supplement your intake of vitamin A, be sure to do so from a plant source rather than a fatty animal source. Rest assured, however, that most people aren't low on A; the fat-soluble form of the vitamin is stored in your liver and usually contains about a two-year supply.

 RDI

Children
2,100–5,000 International Units

Adults
25–50 years: 4,000–5,000 International Units
50+ years: 4,000–6,000 International Units

One of vitamin A's most spectacular characteristics is that it "clones" healthy cells. Often, people with certain types of cancer take vitamin A-based drugs called retinoids, which promote the duplication of healthy cells to ward off the onslaught of unhealthy cells. This works especially well for cancers of tissue linings (except lung cancer) such as the cervix, esophagus, stomach, and intestine. Vitamin A works most efficiently when taken with vitamins B, D, E, and with calcium, phosphorous, and zinc.

 CAUTION!

Like all fat-soluble vitamins, A is highly toxic if taken in large quantities (as little as five to ten times the RDI). Pregnant women who take more than 10,000 IU can harm their fetuses, causing growth retardation or other defects. Signs of an overdose may appear up to six hours after ingestion, including bleeding gums, confusion, hair loss, joint pain, liver damage, dizziness, or double vision.

You may be low in vitamin A if you experience unhealthy bone growth; night blindness; chronic respiratory infections; rough, scaly, dry, and unhealthy skin conditions; vaginal or urinary tract infections; lack of tear secretion; or weight loss. Poor night vision as a result of vitamin A deficiency can lead to blindness.

Smokers who take high doses of vitamin A may actually increase their chance of lung cancer, according to controversial data from the National Institutes for Health. Small amounts are considered safe, but if you smoke, be sure to consult a health care practitioner before taking large doses. Also consult a health practitioner prior to supplementation if you are taking mineral oil, the pill, anticoagulants, antacids, or cholesterol-lowering drugs. Do so also if you have dysfunctions of the kidney, liver, thyroid, or are diabetic.

ANTI-AGING

We are forever in search of the Fountain of Youth or, at the very least, ways to keep our youthful vigor, energy, and looks. Since there is no mystical fountain or magic pill, supplementation—combined with a low-fat, high-fiber diet and exercise—can be quite useful in slowing down the clock.

Antioxidants (vitamins A, C, E, and selenium) are powerful tools for stemming tissue damage from free radicals. Tissue damage occurs throughout our bodies—affecting our bodies internally (brain, cartilage, immune system), as well as externally (skin).

VITAMIN B₁
(Thiamin)

Overall Rating. . . . . *Highly Recommended*

For a healthy heart. . . . . *Highly Recommended*

For optimum brain functioning. . . . . . *Highly Recommended*

To ease motion sickness . . . . *Not Recommended*

If you ever have a scare by experiencing an irregular heartbeat, you'll be reminded of one of the most important reasons to stay up on your vitamin B₁, or thiamin: It keeps your heart muscles flexible and beating to just the right rhythm. This is something we take for granted if everything is in synch. But in those moments when we feel a flutter, a skip, or a thwomp, it becomes very clear that thiamin is essential to life.

Keeping pace with our hearts isn't the only function of thiamin; it also

- acts as a coenzyme to transform carbohydrates into energy
- keeps memory clear and brain functions fully operational
- helps metabolize amino acids into proteins, hormones, and enzymes
- enables absorption of glucose (the sugar from which we get energy)
- converts fatty acids into cortisone and progesterone
- promotes growth
- sustains healthy mucous membranes
- promotes and retains healthy skin
- treats herpes

Although unproven, stocking up on thiamin may also treat motion sickness and depression, act as an insect repellent, decrease pain, and improve appetite.

Thiamin was the first of the B vitamins to be discovered. Shortly after, scientists learned that all the B vitamins depend on each other to properly do what they do both individually and collectively. So, for example, a shortage of B$_{12}$ can actually upset the performance of thiamin—which can throw off the impact of folic acid, and so on. It's extra important, therefore, to get enough of all the B vitamins.

For most of us, getting enough thiamin is easy, since we need so little of it and tend to get enough from our diets. Even so, it is water soluble (meaning our bodies don't store it for a winter's day) and must be replaced daily. You can do this simply by chomping down on sunflower seeds, pork, pecans, oysters, wheat germ, brown rice, raisins, oatmeal, bagels, black beans, green peas, ham, potatoes, chicken, pasta, asparagus, or any product with a label that reads "enriched" (meaning with thiamin, niacin, riboflavin, and iron). That includes breads, cereals, and pastas.

Indeed, if you eat these foods regularly, you probably have plenty of thiamin—unless you drink a lot of alcohol. Alcohol destroys thiamin, and alcoholics often do exhibit deficiencies. In fact, thiamin deficiency is the most common vitamin deficiency in industrialized countries. Even if you drink modestly, it's best not to sip that wine with dinner; rather wait until after the meal. That way, you won't be destroying that little bit of the vitamin that's such a big part of maintaining good health.

Other ways you can unintentionally destroy thiamin is by over-cooking meats or vegetables (it's always best to steam them until their firm but tender), using baking soda in your veggie dishes to keep them looking fresh, eating foods with lots of sulfites or nitrates, or drinking excessive amounts of coffee or tea.

If you fall into one of those categories or if you're over fifty, it's a good idea to supplement.

RDI

Children
0.3–1.5 milligrams

Adults
25–50 years: 1.1–1.6 milligrams
50+ years: 1.0–1.2 milligrams

Supplementation means taking more than the RDI, which is just enough to keep you from getting beriberi, the most extreme symptom of a deficiency. If you're over fifty, you aren't absorbing as much of the vitamin as when you were younger, so you can take considerably more than the RDI. Thiamin is nontoxic, which means you really can't take too much. It's still wise to consult a health care professional for specific doses.

It's also important to increase your thiamin intake if you are consuming lots of carbs. The amount of the vitamin you need will depend on how many carbohydrates you're consuming. You'll also need to supplement if you have a fever or overactive thyroid or are under a lot of stress, to compensate for lost thiamin. If you do supplement, make sure you're getting enough of the other Bs as well as some additional magnesium.

Vegans, women taking oral contraceptives, and the elderly may also benefit from supplementation.

 CAUTION!

Severe alcoholics may experience Wernicke-Korsakoff syndrome, a malfunction of the nerves that, if left unattended, can cause death.

VITAMIN B₂
(Riboflavin)

Overall Rating . . . . *Highly Recommended*

To boost energy . . . . *Highly Recommended*

For proper metabolism . . . . *Highly Recommended*

You know the feeling. It's been a long week. You worked hard. You played even harder. It's the Sunday before your next workweek, and you feel like a semitrailer has hit you.

Energy depletion. If not for riboflavin, or vitamin B_2, we would live in a constant state of energy depletion. That's because this vital vitamin acts as a coenzyme to metabolize fats, proteins, and carbohydrates and turn them into energy. Essentially, if we don't have enough riboflavin in the complex dance involving enzymes, cells, oxygen, and energy release, then we don't have enough energy.

And that's not all. Every cell in our body requires riboflavin to grow and reproduce properly. Our immune system also depends on it for creating the antibodies we need to fight infections. And it plays a significant role in

- promoting and keeping our eyes, skin, hair, and nails healthy
- helping us oxidize amino acids
- contributing to a good memory
- treating carpal tunnel syndrome (along with vitamin B_6 and niacin)
- catalyzing our thyroid function

Riboflavin may even help reduce the chances of getting migraine headaches or cataracts (with supplementation of no more than 10 milligrams per day). When taken with appropriate doses of iron, it reportedly helps with iron deficiencies.

Riboflavin depends on the other B vitamins to work well, just as they depend on riboflavin to carry out their duties. That's why it's so important to make sure you're getting enough of all the Bs. Pyridoxine and niacin, for example, can't do anything right without adequate amounts of riboflavin.

As a water-soluble substance, riboflavin needs to be replaced every day—even though, unlike other water solubles, we do store some of it in the kidney and liver. All the more reason to be mindful of intake: Deficiencies may not show up for several months, since our bodies can pull from their reserve when riboflavin runs low.

But don't wait for symptoms of deficiency to appear. Eat reasonable amounts of foods rich with riboflavin, including beef liver, milk, yogurt, brewer's yeast, cottage cheese, hamburger, almonds, avocados, eggs, ice cream, pork roast, wheat germ, turkey breast, mushrooms, chicken, fish, all those green leafy vegetables, and foods enriched with riboflavin, such as breads, pastas, and cereals.

Unlike other vitamins, riboflavin won't be destroyed by cooking food that contains it, though light will kill it off. That's why milk is best kept in lightproof cartons or slightly colored plastic jugs. Don't worry about the sunshine at your favorite picnic spot, though. It takes a while for the light to do the deed.

If you're a big eater, you actually need more riboflavin than your friends with small appetites do. It shakes down to about .6 milligrams per 1,000 calories. Or, if you're an athlete, you may need more, because the faster you burn energy, the more riboflavin you need. Athletes who supplement may get an added, though unproven benefit: Some claim it helps them train harder and longer and recover more quickly after an especially strenuous workout.

RDI

Children
0.4–1.7 milligrams

Adults
25–50 years: 1.1–1.7 milligrams
50+ years: 1.2–1.4 milligrams

As is often the case, the RDIs reflected here are only the minimum necessary. Athletes, the elderly, vegans, women who take oral contraceptives, diabetics, pregnant and lactating women, people with lactose intolerance, those under excessive stress, or individuals taking certain antidepressant drugs may want to increase their doses. A health care professional can assist with specifics, but since it's nontoxic, doses up to 300 milligrams are typical and up to 1,000 milligrams still safe. High doses may produce bright yellow urine, but that's harmless.

Riboflavin supplements are best taken with a meal and work most effectively when consumed with vitamins B$_6$, C, A, and niacin.

 CAUTION!

Since riboflavin deficiencies are rare, most people don't need to supplement. But if you have these symptoms, you may be low: problems with mucous membranes, cracked lips especially at the corners of the mouth, dry and flaky skin, tearing and red eyes, or anemia. Light sensitivity is also a typical symptom.

People taking anticancer drugs or antibiotics or who drink alcohol may be inhibiting the effects of riboflavin supplements.

VITAMIN B₅
(Pantothenic Acid)

Overall Rating. . . . . *Not Necessary to Supplement*

Remember the days when you had never heard of selenium, St. John's wort, CoQ10, and DHEA? Maybe you still don't know what they're good for (although after reading this book you will). But you've most likely heard of them by now.

Well, pantothenic acid is probably going to spring on us someday just like those other supplements. But not yet. That's because even though we know some of what it does, experts think there are all kinds of other things it can do, too. It will remain in the wings until after conclusive evidence hits the stage, after which stardom will probably strike.

Meanwhile, pantothenic acid plays a role we currently know is critical to our health and well-being. Its primary function is to team up with the other B vitamins (thiamin, riboflavin, and niacin, for example) to turn fat, protein, and carbohydrates into energy. It does this by creating two important enzymes: coenzyme A (CoA) and acyl carrier protein (ACP). These enzymes are also partly responsible for making vitamin D in our bodies. We know, too, that pantothenic acid

- keeps our red blood cells healthy (it's present in all living cells)
- makes hormones
- assists in nerve transmission
- promotes growth
- enables adrenaline to do its job

This little-known vitamin (how often do you wonder if you're getting enough B$_5$?) does all kinds of things we know little about. But time will tell if it actually boosts the immune system; lowers cholesterol; relieves symptoms of lupus, rheumatoid arthritis, and osteoarthritis; helps heal wounds; decreases swelling; wards off fatigue and stress; prevents hair from graying; improves athletic performance; cures allergies; and abates constipation.

If such theories turn into reality, you'll be happy to know that there's virtually no such thing as a pantothenic acid deficiency. That's because it's present in almost every single food we eat. So, vegans and other high-risk individuals don't need to add up how much vitamin B$_5$ they're missing to figure out how much to supplement. Nor does anyone else.

Some of the foods richest in vitamin B$_5$ are: salmon, yogurt, baked potatoes, cooked mushrooms, lentils, chicken liver, chicken legs, lima beans, eggs, corn, milk, beef liver, and on and on and on.

The only warning about food preparation is that when you freeze meat, thaw it, then cook it, half of the pantothenic acid is lost.

Shouldn't matter, though, as long as you're getting enough of all your other B vitamins. Remember—they all depend on one another to fulfill their destinies.

 ## RECOMMENDED USAGE

There is no RDI, since there aren't any deficiencies (except for people who are starving themselves). What is believed, however, is that we need between 4 and 10 milligrams per day. An easy deal, since that's covered even in low-cal diets.

Supplements are therefore unnecessary—especially if you simply want reassurance that you have enough CoA and ACP. Trust us on this: You do have enough. What supplements might be good for—and *might* is the key word here—is to lower cholesterol. But think about it: There are so many other nutritional supplements and vitamins (i.e., niacin) that positively do the trick, it seems silly to take a chance on a B$_5$ supplement.

 CAUTION!

There are no known deficiencies unless under controlled circumstances. Supplements are nontoxic, since this is a water-soluble substance that will be excreted if it's not needed.

VITAMIN B$_6$
(Pyridoxine)

Overall Rating. . . . . *Highly Recommended*

To boost metabolism . . . . *Highly Recommended*

To prevent water retention . . . . *Recommended*

To aid the immune system . . . . *Highly Recommended*

To boost brain functioning. . . . . *Highly Recommended*

Ever heard of ascorbic acid? Most people have. How about folic acid? Probably so. What about niacin and riboflavin? Yep. But when it comes to pyridoxine, the vast majority most likely haven't ever heard of it, much less know that it's just as important and critical to our health as any of those more famous vitamins.

Pyridoxine is actually one of three substances that make up vitamin B$_6$. Pyridoxine itself is found mostly in plant sources, while pyridoxamine and pyridoxal, the other two substances, are typically found in animal foods. Each basically covers the same biological activity as the others do, so they are all lumped together and simply called pyridoxine.

And just what does pyridoxine do? For starters, it performs over sixty different functions as a coenzyme, such as metabolizing protein and amino acids so we can draw energy from them. In addition, makes antibodies so we stay healthy and produces red blood cells (hemoglobin), hormones, neurotransmitters, and prostaglandin. All that, and pyridoxine is also thought to be essential to

❦ keeping homocysteine levels in check so we don't have hardening of the arteries, which, in the end, causes heart attacks and strokes

- ❦ ensuring a normal, functioning brain
- ❦ maintaining a healthy and active immune system
- ❦ properly converting tryptophan into niacin
- ❦ synthesizing hydrochloric acid and magnesium
- ❦ effectively absorbing vitamin B$_{12}$
- ❦ eliminating unnecessary water from our bodies
- ❦ preventing skin and nerve disorders

Some of the benefits of supplementing vitamin B$_6$ include the reduction of muscle spasms, numbness in extremities, and cramps in legs; relieving some asthmatic symptoms; lowering blood pressure; treating certain diabetic conditions; working as a natural diuretic; and easing allergic reactions to MSG.

We still don't know whether pyridoxine supplements can actually do other great things, but there have been positive results in some cases. Try supplements to ease symptoms of PMS, morning sickness, carpal tunnel syndrome, melanoma, and depression, and if you're diabetic, talk to your doctor about how it can reduce your need for insulin. It may also ward off the nasty side effects associated with cancer-treating drugs and has been used to treat several types of mental illness.

Now that you know all about this busy B, it may surprise you to learn that deficiencies are fairly common. An odd fact, given that B$_6$ is found in almost every food we eat, even though many foods, like most fruits and vegetables, contain only tiny amounts. But remember: If you're deficient in one of the B vitamins, the functions of all B vitamins are impaired. So forage through your fridge and cupboards and pull out these B$_6$-rich foods: brewer's yeast, wheat bran, wheat germ, turkey, peanuts, molasses, bananas, some cereals, eggs, brussel sprouts, halibut, avocados, pork chops, baked potatoes, roast beef, cantaloupes, beef liver, chicken, canned tuna, salmon, cottage cheese, milk, spinach, grapefruit, and lima beans.

Beware that freezing vegetables, overcooking, and canning foods pretty much depletes their pyridoxine, so do what you can to avoid these.

 RDI

Children
0.3–2 milligrams

Adults
25–50 years: 1.6–2 milligrams
50+ years: 2 milligrams

Since pyridoxine is so integral to the breakdown of protein, it stands to reason—and it's true—that the amount you need is really determined by how much protein you eat. For every gram of protein you consume, .016 milligrams of pyridoxine is needed to break it down. Experts estimate that men consume around 125 grams of protein, resulting in the need for approximately 2 milligrams of pyridoxine. Women evidently eat slightly less protein, so they can get away with about 1.6 milligrams.

A multivitamin can provide adequate amounts of this precious B, but if you're looking to treat symptoms of a condition, you'll need more.

People most susceptible to deficiencies include pregnant or breastfeeding women, those on birth control pills or estrogen, bodybuilders who eat a lot of protein, vegans, alcoholics, people taking steroids or antibiotics, individuals who have kidney stones or Down's syndrome, and those who take certain drugs for asthma.

Pyridoxine is water soluble, so it's safe to supplement up to about 500 milligrams. Unlike other water-soluble substances, however, *pyridoxine is very toxic when taken in larger doses.* Be sure to work with a health care professional if you decide to supplement for conditions that require large doses.

 CAUTION!

Deficiencies are recognized in those with a weak immune system, anemia, oily and scaly skin, mental confusion, and nervousness.

Toxic reactions include tingling of extremities, which can lead to irreparable nerve damage if left untreated. Most often, simply discontinuing the supplement will solve the problem. Overdoses may also cause kidney stones.

Do not supplement if you're on drugs for Parkinson's disease or epilepsy. Consult a doctor prior to supplementing to treat serious conditions.

VITAMIN C
(Ascorbic Acid)

Overall Rating . . . . *Highly Recommended*

To repair damaged tissue . . . . *Highly Recommended*

To heal wounds and broken bones . . . *Highly Recommended*

To protect against cancer . . . . *Recommended*

To protect against heart disease . . . . . *Highly Recommended*

To lower cholesterol and

blood pressure . . . . *Highly Recommended*

For treating urinary tract infections . . . *Highly Recommended*

To increase sperm count . . . . *Recommended*

It's an American tradition: Sneeze a few times, sniffle once, and reach for the Cs. Ironically, most people probably don't know that science hasn't yet proven vitamin C prevents or cures colds. Even so, the average health-conscious person believes that the king of vitamins can combat the aches and pains of the common cold. And the truth is that taking the vitamin while sick does make people feel better faster. The bottom line? Both the upstairs and downstairs cupboards are chock-full of it.

Which is fine, because what we know for sure about this vitamin is that it's very good for us in all kinds of ways, and it's basically nontoxic. Numerous clinical, experimental, and population studies have shown that vitamin C has lots of benefits, including

   .❀ promoting collagen formation, which connects tissues, adheres muscles to bones, repairs damaged tissue, and heals wounds and broken bones

- protecting against cancer, heart disease, and cataracts and helping treat diabetes
- contributing to red blood cell production in bone marrow
- integrating proteins, carbohydrates, and fats in our systems
- lowering cholesterol, blood pressure, and the incidence of stroke and kidney disease
- keeping blood vessels strong
- building healthy capillaries, gums, and teeth
- helping synthesize hormonal functions, including that of thyroid
- helping with absorption of folic acid, iron, and calcium
- supporting amino acid metabolism
- treating anemia, scurvy, urinary tract infections, and iron deficiencies

A critical role this vitamin plays is that of Most Important Antioxidant. We know free radicals are responsible for heart disease, cancer, and other illnesses. We also know antioxidants kill off free radicals, leaving us healthier and living longer. Vitamin C is, in essence, the commander in chief of the artillery used to wipe out free radicals. So widespread is its effect, some experts believe that if you supplement your diet with nothing more than vitamin C, you'll be doing most of what's necessary to stave off heart disease, cancer, high blood pressure, and the physical stresses related to pollution and other environmental toxins.

And there's more: If you're feeling a little bloated, vitamin C works as a natural laxative. Or, if you're a man with a low sperm count, increase your Cs and watch the count rise! Not only will your sperm count benefit, the man who takes it may also live longer than his buddies who don't.

Although conclusive supporting evidence is lacking, many health care professionals use vitamin C to treat (rather than prevent) cancer, arthritis, cataracts, and hay fever or to prevent colds and blood clots.

Given the hale and hearty effects of the vitamin, it's a good thing there are so many foods that contain it. Orange juice is probably the most typical source, but all citrus fruits have an abundance. So does cantaloupe, collards, broccoli, peppers, green leafy vegetables, cabbage, guava, mango, papaya, kiwi, strawberries, rose hips, tomatoes, and watercress. Beware, however, that overcooking can destroy a good bit of the vitamin C in these foods. So eat them raw, or go for al dente.

 RDI

Children
35–60 milligrams

Adults
25+ years: 60–200 milligrams

Smokers, heavy drinkers, women on birth control pills, and people who live in cities have less vitamin C in their systems than the rest of us. That's because those nefarious agents—nicotine, alcohol, and carbon monoxide—actually destroy or inhibit the vitamin. Eating plenty of vitamin C–rich foods is vital for such people, but supplementation is a surefire way of getting all the Cs they need.

Since vitamin C is water soluble, what we ingest only remains in our system for about four hours before being absorbed or excreted. We can take between 1,000 and 4,000 milligrams a day before experiencing diarrhea—nature's way of telling us we've had enough. It all depends on how badly we need the supplement and how sensitive we are to it.

If you decide to supplement, take the vitamin with magnesium, bioflavonoids, and calcium. If you use a lot of aspirin, you'll need more than if you don't, since the two don't complement each other. And, if you're also taking ginseng, wait three hours before or after you've ingested it before downing your Cs.

 CAUTION!

It's easy to get enough vitamin C, and scurvy, the most common symptom of a deficiency, is rare these days. But some people eat way too much fast food, and they forget to take their supplements. For them, deficiencies could manifest as muscle weakness, bruises, swollen or bleeding gums, loose teeth, depression, digestive problems, nosebleeds, and anemia. A less obvious result of too little C is that your body won't be able to flush itself of cholesterol or fight off infectious diseases. Free radicals will have a ball as a C-deprived body hosts them to a feast of fatal "attractions."

Unlikely overdoses can result as kidney stones, dizziness, fainting, and vomiting.

Consult your health care professional if these symptoms occur, of if you are planning to supplement and you have gout or sickle cell anemia or if you are on anticoagulants, aspirin, barbiturates, estrogen, cortisone, or birth control pills.

VITAMIN D

Overall Rating. . . . . *Highly Recommended*

For healthy bones and teeth . . . . *Highly Recommended*

To prevent colds . . . . *Recommended*

To reduce symptoms of menopause. . . *Recommended*

To protect against cancer . . . . *Recommended*

Vitamin D is often called the sunshine vitamin, but a more accurate nickname might be the "bone-enhancer" vitamin. That's because its primary function is to assist with the absorption of calcium and phosphorous, which ultimately helps build healthy bones and teeth and maintain bone density. It also has hormonal-like effects on mineral absorption, bone mineralization, and secretion.

But like most other vitamins, this one offers plenty of other benefits: It can help protect against colon and rectal cancers, treat psoriasis, increase muscle strength and, when taken with vitamin C, prevent colds, treat conjunctivitis, and help our bodies absorb vitamin A. "It is also believed it can improve symptoms for postmenopausal women or women on estrogen replacement therapy," states Christiane Northrup, M.D., author of *Women's Bodies, Women's Wisdom* and past president of the American Holistic Medical Association.

It's easy to get enough vitamin D, since there's plenty of it in different foods, and—here comes the sun—we can get it simply by being outside on a beautiful day!

If you are fair-skinned, for example, and take a ten-minute walk on a sunny day in a T-shirt, your body will produce enough vitamin D for the entire day. How? By absorbing ultraviolet rays from the sun. They travel to the liver, undergo a chemical change, then travel through the bloodstream to the kidney, where they transform into dihydroxy vitamin D.

If you're dark-skinned, you'll need to walk for about three hours for the same thing to happen. The pigment in darker-skinned people blocks out the ultraviolet rays that are essential to this metamorphosis. Either way, don't worry about the sun giving you an overdose; our bodies simply stop converting sunshine into this essential vitamin when it has had enough.

But beware—if you're wearing sunblock or a long-sleeved shirt or coat, or if it's cloudy or smoggy out, you'll have to find another source for your vitamin D. Those elements block out the rays that produce the phenomenon.

You can also get your vitamin D from the foods you eat. The best sources include

- seafood, such as canned sardines, fresh mackerel, cod liver oil, herring, salmon, and shrimp
- fortified milk or dairy products: butter, cream
- egg yolks
- fortified cereals
- cooked liver

Vitamin D is fat soluble, meaning it stays in the body for longer periods of time than water-soluble vitamins do. It is stored in human and animal fat and liver. That's why eating fish or animal liver provides such high doses. If you are low on vitamin D, consider an oral supplement so you don't eat too much fatty food.

 RDI

Children
200–400 IU

Women

25–50 years:	200–400 IU
50+ years:	400–600 IU
Nursing mothers:	200–500 IU

Men

25–50 years:	200–400 IU
50+ years:	400–600 IU

 CAUTION!

This is the most toxic of all vitamins. It only takes 2,000 IU per day, or five times the RDI, to be toxic in children. Adult overdoses can cause permanent damage by increasing blood calcium levels, leading to calcium deposits in the kidneys, heart, and other tissues.

Symptoms of overdose include severe and constant headache, diarrhea, and/or nausea.

Deficiencies are rare these days, but if you don't get enough vitamin D, your bones will lose their calcium, protein, and minerals, creating osteomalacia. Meanwhile, your blood pressure could go up, and you might be setting yourself up for some serious osteoporosis.

If your kids don't get enough of this essential vitamin, their bones won't develop properly from lack of calcium, and they could develop rickets.

If you decide to supplement your diet with D, consult your doctor first if you're taking antacids, anticonvulsants, barbiturates, and high doses of calcium, mineral oil, or diuretics.

MULTIVITAMINS

The need for supplementation stems from the fact that, try as we may, most of us do not consistently eat a diet that is well-balanced and reflects the optimal levels and ranges of nutrients. Even for those of us who do a remarkable job of eating well, factors such as the soil vegetables are grown in and the way produce is stored and shipped can rob food of vital nutrients.

As you read the labels of different multivitamin products, you will find variations in the nutrient levels, as well as varying levels of quality. Your best bet is to buy from established and reputable companies; they tend to be more trustworthy than smaller manufacturers. Although you may end up paying a bit more, a well-known company is a guarantee you're getting the real thing.

Be aware that some of these—like those all-important antioxidants—are often best taken separately, not in a multivitamin. It's more cost-effective to take individually than in a multiple formula especially vitamins E and C.

Here then are the recommended ingredients and dosages in a multivitamin:

- Vitamin A (beta-carotene)—5,000–25,000 IU
- Vitamin D—100–400 IU
- Vitamin E (d-alpha tocopherol)—100–800 IU
- Vitamin K (phytonadione)—60–300 micrograms
- Vitamin C (ascorbic acid)—100–1,000 milligrams
- Vitamin B_1 (thiamin)—10–100 milligrams
- Vitamin B_{12} (riboflavin)—10–50 milligrams
- Niacin—10–100 milligrams

- Vitamin B$_6$ (pyridoxine)—25–100 milligrams
- Biotin—100–300 micrograms
- Folate (folic acid)—400 micrograms
- Vitamin B$_{12}$—400 micrograms
- Choline—10–100 milligrams
- Boron—1–6 milligrams
- Calcium—400–1,500 milligrams
- Chromium—200 micrograms
- Copper—3 milligrams
- Iodine—150 micrograms
- Iron—10–50 milligrams
- Magnesium—400 milligrams
- Molybdenum—100 micrograms
- Potassium—300 milligrams
- Selenium—200 micrograms
- Zinc—30 micrograms

Often multivitamin combinations are formulated for specific purposes, such as aiding sleep or weight loss, enhancing immune function, raising energy levels, or during pregnancy. Consult with your doctor before deciding which multivitamin combination is the most appropriate for you.

         🙢 🙢 🙢

VITAMIN E

Overall Rating . . . . *Highly Recommended*

To decrease the risk of cancer . . . . *Recommended*

To improve male fertility . . . . *Highly Recommended*

To boost the immune system . . . . *Highly Recommended*

For menopausal symptoms . . . . *Highly Recommended*

For breast conditions . . . . *Recommended*

If vitamin C is the commander-in-chief of the army that protects us from free radicals, vitamin E could be called a five-star general. You remember what free radicals are: the out-of-control molecules that cause oxidation in our bodies, resulting in cancer, heart disease, and other life-threatening conditions. Vitamin E has just the necessary defense mechanisms to keep these radicals from wreaking oxidation havoc, especially on vitamin A, selenium, and some essential amino acids.

So critical is its role as "star" antioxidant that recent studies reveal vitamin E to be largely responsible for maintaining a healthy heart and even healing an unhealthy one. This is because it keeps LDL (bad cholesterol) from oxidizing and clogging up the arteries that lead to the heart (known as hardening of the arteries). So, even if you already have heart disease, taking between 400 and 800 IUs per day can actually help unclog the passages (it helps, it doesn't cure). And, if you've had surgery to clean out your arteries, regular doses of vitamin E can help you recover faster and keep them clean longer. Talk about getting to the heart of the matter!

Not only that, but vitamin E is busy with other projects, too. At the same time it's policing the LDL in your arteries, it's also

* lowering incidence of mouth, throat, and esophagus cancer
* repelling the agents that create some lung cancers, especially from environmental toxins
* decreasing the risk of breast and cervical cancer in women
* protecting against colon cancer in men
* improving male fertility
* boosting the immune system, especially in people over sixty-five
* acting as an anticoagulant
* assisting enzymes to do what they do best
* relieving tender fibrocystic breasts, as well as some menopausal symptoms in women
* easing leg cramps

That's a list of what we know for sure. But there are other jobs this vitamin may perform. For example: slowing the effects of sickle-cell anemia, Alzheimer's, and Parkinson's disease; preventing cataracts; controlling blood sugar levels in diabetics; speeding the recovery of external cuts, burns, or wounds; erasing scars or stretch marks; beefing up athletic performance—even enhancing sexual performance!

And here's something to think about during sleepless nights: People with cancer consistently have low levels of vitamin E. Researchers aren't sure yet if the low levels of vitamin E caused the cancer or if the low levels are a result of the cancer. Since we know the vitamin helps prevent some cancers, it may be wise to supplement, just in case those low levels really are related to the incidence of disease.

So how does this super substance work? Vitamin E can be broken down into two different categories: tocopherols and tocotrienols. Ever since we've discovered what vitamin E does so well, we've credited the dominant form of tocopherol, or alpha-tocopherol, for most of the good work. That's where the majority of antioxidant warriors reside, which is why the vitamin is so effective.

The latest updates reveal something new, however. In 1997, studies showed that what makes up tocotrienol may, in fact, be a stronger antioxidant and the one responsible for lowering cholesterol and reducing abnormal blood clotting. This form of the vitamin also reportedly reduces tumors in women with breast cancer.

What does all this mean to you? Very simply that you need both forms of it. Wheat germ is a terrific source of tocopherols; rice bran provides the most tocotrienols. But who wants to meet someone at a nice restaurant for a big bowl of those? Sure, you could add other vitamin E–rich foods to your meal, like sunflower oil or seeds, hazelnuts, almonds, almond oil, peanut butter, fortified cereals, avocados, mangoes, or asparagus. But it would take an awful lot to get the amounts necessary to benefit your heart and lower cholesterol. The answer? Supplementation, of course.

 RDI

Children
3–10 milligrams, or 4.5–15 IU

Adults
25–50 years: 8–10 milligrams, or 12–15 IU
50+ years: 8–10 milligrams, or 12–15 IU

As is typical for RDIs, these numbers reflect the minimum necessary so as not to be deficient. They don't come close to what you need to reap the benefits of a healthier heart or a strong antioxidant army. As a general rule, for the preventative protection this vitamin provides, take anywhere from 100 to 800 IUs per day. It's hard to overdose on vitamin E, since we excrete whatever we don't need, probably within a day. What we do need is stored in fatty tissues, the liver, heart, muscles, testes, uterus, blood, and adrenal and pituitary glands. Even so, it's always smart to work with a health care practitioner on specific doses.

For the best tocopherol form of the vitamin, choose a supplement with "d-alpha-tocopherol" on the label. For the best tocotrienols form, ask a nutritionist. Always take these supplements with a meal.

When taking vitamin E supplements, keep these pointers in mind: Doses are not universal. Small people need less and big people need more. People who eat a lot of fat need more. People who eat very little fat may need to eat a bit more of it for vitamin E to work effectively. It's best when taken with

- a small amount of fat
- vitamin C
- beta-carotene
- vitamin A (though if you take too much E, it can block the functions of A)

 CAUTION!

Unlike other fat-soluble vitamins, this one is basically nontoxic.

Deficiencies are rare, but symptoms manifest as age (liver) spots, lethargy, decreased sexual performance, and sometimes nerve damage.

People with cystic fibrosis, iron deficiencies, Crohn's disease, an overactive thyroid, or liver disease or those on blood-thinning drugs should consult a doctor prior to supplementation.

VITAMIN K

Overall Rating . . . . *Recommended*

To stimulate blood clotting. . . . . *Highly Recommended*

To reduce morning sickness
in pregnancy . . . . *Recommended*

For treating skin conditions . . . . *Recommended*

Ask a new mother what vitamin K does, and she may not have a clear answer, but she could very possibly have a strange, unpleasant reaction to the question—and not even know why. Here's a clue from the doctors at the University of Colorado Medical Center: In the ecstatic fog that envelops a woman after giving birth, she'll watch as someone injects her precious newborn with a shot of vitamin K. The infant will wail, the mother will wince and reach for her baby with teary eyes. In that moment, she may, perhaps for the first time, experience the primal need to protect her young.

Even though the incident was discomforting, injecting a baby with vitamin K actually supports a mother's instinct to protect. That's because newborns don't have the intestinal bacteria that produces the vitamin, putting them at risk of hemorrhaging if, for any reason, they start to bleed. "While this isn't the case in all newborns, vitamin K is considered a helpful adjunct in many natal units today," explains pediatrician Lendon Smith of Portland, Oregon.

In addition, the *British Medical Journal* reports that many pediatrician consider oral vitamin K as good or better than an injection.

This fat-soluble vitamin is the ingredient that produces the substances that clot our blood. Deficiencies are rare, since our intestinal bacteria create about half of what we need, while eating foods rich with the vitamin provides the rest.

But helping us to recover after a quick nick on the thumb while chopping vegetables isn't the only thing vitamin K can do. It also directs calcium to our bones and ensures the bones absorb it so they can develop normally, stay strong, and prevent osteoporosis. It also prevents internal bleeding and reduces extreme menstrual flow.

Recent studies from the University of California at Santa Cruz indicate that, taken with vitamin C, vitamin K can greatly reduce morning sickness in pregnant women. It may also retard osteoporosis, reduce tumors, kill cancer cells, and treat skin conditions such as spider veins, broken capillaries, bruises, sun-damaged skin, and postoperative scars.

Getting enough of this life-saving vitamin is easy since, as mentioned, a good bit of it is produced within our intestines. And the foods that provide us with the rest are pretty delicious, including peas, ham, green beans, yogurt, egg yolk, soybean and fish liver oils, green tea leaves, strawberries, turnips, lettuce, cabbage, spinach, broccoli, asparagus, and seaweed.

 RDI

The RDI for vitamin K depends on the weight of each individual. The listings here reflect average doses.

Children
5–140 micrograms (averaging 30–60 micrograms)

Adults
25–50 years: 5–140 micrograms (averaging 60–80 micrograms)
50+ years: 5–140 micrograms (averaging 70–80 micrograms)

CAUTION!

Deficiencies of vitamin K are most common in people with chronic gastrointestinal disorders or in those unable to absorb fat. Deficiencies are often caused by long-term use of antibiotics (since they kill off the good bacteria in our intestines, from which vitamin K is produced), eating too few green leafy vegetables or other foods rich in the vitamin, extreme exposure to severe air pollution, or having liver disease (since a healthy liver is required to help make substances that clot blood).

Signs of deficiencies are:

- hemorrhaging
- liver and gallbladder disease
- disease of the intestinal tract
- nosebleeds
- blood in the urine
- bruises
- failure to grow in infants
- (possibly) excessive diarrhea

Each of our bodies regulates how much vitamin K it makes and cannot overdose itself. An overdose can occur only by taking too much synthetic vitamin K. So if you take vitamin K supplements, be sure to take correct amounts. Also beware that supplementing with large doses of vitamin K may actually cause bleeding. Symptoms of an overdose include jaundice, brain damage, and impaired liver damage.

Consult a health practitioner before supplementating just prior to surgery or if you are taking mineral oil, cholesterol-lowering drugs, aspirin, anticoagulants, excessive caffeine, laxatives, penicillin or other antibiotics, or prednizone.

WILD YAM

Overall Rating. . . . . *Recommended*

For alleviating menopausal symptoms . . . . . . *Recommended*

No one can argue that the yams we gobble down during the holiday season are good for us. They're packed with vitamin A, which contains beta-carotene, an essential element for good vision. But there's a different kind of yam, wild yam—often called Mexican wild yam—that isn't even a remote relative to the yams we know. Even so, it's at least as valuable as the substance we're more familiar with—especially if you're a menopausal woman.

Wild yam is a vine that grows in central and southern North America. It's been called "devil's bones" since it resembles a skeleton. But there's nothing scary about this plant. Rather, it's packed with all kinds of useful properties. Most notably, it has a chemical structure that is identical to that of progesterone, an essential hormone created in a woman's body.

Because of this remarkable chemical compound, wild yam is nature's perfect answer to progesterone replacement. The need for more progesterone can occur before menopausal symptoms occur, as well as during and after them. The key to understanding if you need progesterone is ovulation: If you ovulate, you create progesterone. If you don't ovulate, you don't create it. You can still menstruate and not ovulate, which is when you might need it prior to menopause.

Most typically, however, women need progesterone once they start to experience those hot flashes and mood swings so commonly associated with menopause. This is when the body stops manufacturing estrogen. Mainstream medicine commonly prescribes estrogen replacement therapies (ERT) for menopausal women, but sadly, there can be devastating side effects after several years of using these therapies. The most common side effect of ERT is excessive growth that may lead to cancer. What's more, when ERTs are employed, the treatment completely dismisses the important role of progesterone in the overall health of a woman.

Most of the studies conducted by today's leaders in menopause therapies conclude that natural progesterone is a good, safe way to supplement during menopause. Unlike synthetic hormones (or equine hormones, as in the commonly prescribed drug Premarin), natural progresterone cleanly binds with a woman's own estrogens, assisting her body to perform what it does naturally, says John Lee, M.D., author of *What Your Doctor May Not Tell You About Menopause*.

A menopausal woman's most serious threat is osteoporosis, since estrogen is what prevents bone loss. But consider this: Progesterone stimulates bone formation—the other, just as viable approach to protecting against osteoporosis. But there's one enormous benefit. Unlike synthetic forms of estrogen or progesterone (called progestins), there are no known side effects when using yam-based progesterone creams.

That's why we salute the valuable ingredients found in this vine. Simply apply ½ to 1 teaspoon of yam-based progesterone cream to the abdomen, inner thighs, arms, or face, and it will flow directly to your bloodstream to help build new bone tissue. This is the preferred method of application, since the blood stream is the natural residence for hormones.

Many women these days are choosing not to use ERTs because of the increased incidence of breast and uterine cancer that can result. Instead, they're turning to yam-based progesterone creams.

Augmenting with vitamins C and D, exercising, and eating a healthy diet have helped diminish the discomforts of menopause.

Taken in the form of a tincture or decoction, wild yam also helps relieve symptoms of

- rheumatism
- irritable bowel syndrome
- labor or postpartum pain
- menstrual cramps
- urinary tract infections
- kidney imbalances
- colic
- stomach cramps
- nausea
- vomiting
- vaginal dryness

 RECOMMENDED USAGE

There is no RDI for wild yam.

Children

Not advised for children. Administer only under the advice of a doctor or health practitioner.

Adults

If you're trying to ease the inflammation and joint pain associated with rheumatism, take twenty-five drops twice daily.

As rule, adults can take up to 1 teaspoon of the tincture three times a day.

If you're taking a decoction, you can take up to one cup three times a day.

If you're using wild yam cream intravaginally, speak with your practitioner to make sure you're getting the purest form. And check with your doctor to make sure this is the optimal therapy for your particular needs.

As always, it's best to work with a health care professional to determine specific doses for the conditions you're treating.

 CAUTION!

Since wild yam has hormonal properties, be mindful that it will act as such in your body. If you have any hormonal imbalances, consult a doctor before supplementing with this herb.

WITCH HAZEL
(*Hamamelis virginiana*)

Overall Rating. . . . . *Highly Recommended*

**For healing cuts, and other
skin repair**. *Highly Recommended*

Is it a cartoon character? There's Broom Hilda, and then there's Witch Hazel, right? Well, yes, but the difference is that the former lives playfully between book covers, while the latter is kept in medicine cabinets around the world.

First used by the Native Americans, the American witch hazel plant is a small deciduous tree or shrub with twisted bark and twisted yellow flowers. All that twisting and turning can be broken down to three basic chemical compounds: tannic acid, gallic acid, and volatile oil. Thanks to those three ingredients, witch hazel is an effective and soothing astringent, which can help relieve uncomfortable skin conditions, including

- sunburn
- insect bites or stings
- bruises
- abrasions
- rash from poison ivy or oak
- oily skin
- diaper rash
- eczema
- bed sores

Witch hazel is also useful as an aftershave, or when diluted and dropped into tired eyes, or when added to a hot bath to relax sore or aching muscles. Also, taking a witch hazel steam bath can help break up phlegm from colds or coughs.

 ## RECOMMENDED USAGE

There is no RDI for witch hazel.

You can find witch hazel in grocery stores, drugstores, or health food stores in just about any town in the country. It's widely accepted as soothing to the skin, it's inexpensive, and it's safe. It's sold mostly as a liquid tincture.

If you can find some raw bark and leaves, make a tea by placing 1 tablespoon of the bark and leaves into 1 pint of boiling water. Let steep for forty-five minutes. The tea is useful as a gargle for sore throats or as a tonic for diarrhea, hemorrhoids, or ulcers. If you choose to drink the tea, work with a health care professional to make sure you are ingesting the right amount.

To treat bruises or sprains, consider making witch hazel ice cubes and applying the ice to the affected area.

Use diluted tincture for a mouthwash or as a douche for vaginitis.

 ## CAUTION!

Witch hazel is considered safe, but again, if you decide to ingest it, work with a health care practitioner first.

YUCCA

Overall Rating . . . . *Recommended*

For treating symptoms of arthritis . . . *Highly Recommended*
To slow the growth of tumors . . . . . . *Recommended*

Yucca plants live in the desert. A member of the *Liliaceae* family, they're, in fact, everywhere in the desert. They come in all different shapes and sizes, from small scrubby shrubs to imposing trees that stand up to 60 feet high. You may be familiar with the Joshua tree (after all, there is a national park named in its honor), which scatters across much of the Southern California desert. Even if you aren't aware of them—or fond of their sharp, cactuslike appearance—you might be glad to know of them if you ever have trouble with arthritis.

The National Arthritis Medical Clinic, located in Southern California, took an isolated property from the yucca plant called saponin and administered it to people with severe symptoms of arthritis. Their preliminary studies found that saponin had positive therapeutic effects on most of the participants. This good news was reported in *The Journal of Applied Nutrition.*

Other studies reported in both *Oncology* and *Growth* concur that yucca plants can offer us another, critically important benefit. The fresh flowers of the yucca plant contain an antitumor agent and can therefore strongly inhibit the growth of tumors. Laboratory studies also show that the fresh flower can help treat melanoma and leukemia.

RECOMMENDED USAGE

There is no RDI for yucca.

Children

Not advised for children. Administer only under the advice of a doctor or health practitioner.

Adults

Capsules

One 100 milligram-capsule up to three times daily.

Tincture

Three drops in an 8-ounce glass of water three times daily.

If you suffer from arthritis and want to try yucca to relieve pain, take four to six tablets daily (or 2 to 4 grams three times a day) on an empty stomach.

 CAUTION!

Yucca is nontoxic and has no apparent side effects.

If you have a lump or tumor, consult a physician before attempting to treat it yourself. And, as always, work with your doctor so you don't interfere with existing treatments.

ZINC

Overall Rating . . . . *Highly Recommended*

For relieving cold symptoms . . . . *Highly Recommended*

To counter benign prostatic
hyperplasia . . . . *Recommended*

When you've got a bad cold and you're downing vitamin C, drinking gallons of juice, inhaling a tree's worth of eucalyptus, and weeding through every box of tissue in the house, don't forget to take a few zinc lozenges, too. If you do, you'll get over the cold faster. That's because zinc nudges the thymus gland to direct our bodies to create all infection-fighting agents, thus activating our immune system. Plus, zinc is actually part of superoxide dismutase, which is an antioxidant. What does all this mean? Zinc helps us to feel better.

Boosting our immune system and helping us get over a cold is one thing. But zinc helps us in lots of other ways by

- synthesizing RNA and DNA so our cells can divide, repair themselves, and grow
- teaming up with at least 200 different enzymes so they can do what they do
- making the hormones that control growth
- providing the right mix of what makes healthy testosterone
- making sure we have the correct acid-alkaline balance
- contributing to the production of insulin
- enabling muscles to contract
- aiding in the metabolism of carbohydrates, fats, and proteins

Zinc is found in our bones, skin, hair, nails, eyes, and in the prostate and testes. It makes sense, then, that zinc is largely what helps heal wounds and psoriasis; promote strong and healthy skin, hair, and nails; increase sperm count; reverse male infertility; and treat or prevent prostate problems.

Fact is, men who have benign prostate hypertrophy (BPH) generally have low levels of zinc. Supplementation can ease the symptoms. Healthy men over fifty might consider taking zinc as a regular part of their diet, since it can keep prostate troubles at bay. Meanwhile, it can decrease cholesterol deposits that might be building up, which could eventually lead to heart trouble.

Younger men who have low sperm counts can multiply the numbers just by increasing their intake of zinc. And if there's a problem with impotence, it may even correct that in conjunction with vitamin B_6.

If you're reproductive centers are working well, but your olfactory senses are on the blink, curiously, zinc can help restore a sense of smell and taste to whomever may have lost it.

It also keeps us from absorbing lead and other environmental toxins. And although we don't know for sure that it fights these diseases, it is true that people with AIDS and cancer exhibit low levels of zinc.

Other speculative attributes include regulating menses, encouraging recovery from anorexia, and treating schizophrenia.

By now, you realize that getting enough of this substance is pretty important. And a lot of us don't. Especially vegans, who don't eat animal products; diabetics; pregnant and breastfeeding women; those over fifty; people with sickle-cell anemia; and those who enjoy the cocktail hour. So listen up!

It's hard to get enough zinc from food, since we only absorb 10 percent from what we eat. Even if we ate all the right foods, including oysters, chicken, ground beef, wheat germ, white beans, yogurt, lentils, chickpeas, beef liver, almonds, black beans, turkey,

Swiss cheese, pecans, oatmeal, and cashews (notice there isn't a single fruit in here), we'd still run short. That's because most of the foods are grown in nutrient-poor soil with little zinc in it, and on top of that, cooking virtually destroys what's left.

So getting a good supplement is paramount. That's easy when you get it in the form of zinc gluconate (easy to absorb), zinc picolinate, zinc citrate, or zinc monomethionate. Pass over the zinc sulfate, though, since it could upset your stomach. And take the supplement with a meal that isn't high in fiber.

 RDI

Children
5–12 milligrams

Adults
25–50 years: 12–15 milligrams
50+ years: 12–15 milligrams
Lozenges
For colds and flus, a recommended dosage is six to ten lozenges daily, as needed.

We've said it before, we'll say it again: The RDI is the smallest amount required before a deficiency kicks in. Optimum doses are more realistically between 30 and 50 micrograms for adults.

Take a little more zinc if you're supplementing with lots of vitamin B_6.

Zinc works best when taken with vitamin A (zinc and A are old friends, since one of zinc's jobs is to escort the vitamin A that's stored in the liver and take it to where it's needed in the body), calcium, and phosphorous. Take additional copper with larger doses.

CAUTION!

Serious deficiencies are rare, but those that do occur can generally be corrected with supplementation. Children who don't grow properly may be deficient. Other symptoms include slow sexual development, delayed healing of wounds, skin problems, hair loss, and frequent infections.

Taking more than 150 milligrams a day could be toxic. Overdosing on zinc can block the absorption of copper, calcium, and iron and inhibit the immune system. It's difficult to overdose, however, without immediate repercussions, such as vomiting and diarrhea.

Pregnant women should make sure they get enough zinc, since low levels can lead to toxemia, which could threaten the pregnancy.

BUYER BEWARE:
Tips for Choosing a Supplement

Because supplementation has recently become such big business, there are many, many supplement companies that sell vast lines of products. Unfortunately, some of these companies even sell supplements that contain none of the active ingredients! For example, in a 1997 analysis of fifteen different brands of glucosamine and chondroitin supplements by the University of Maryland, researchers discovered that the amount found in the samples varied significantly from the amount printed on the label in nearly half of the brands.

How does a concerned consumer make sure they're getting the right thing? Obviously each of these companies can't be evaluated individually, and new ones keep springing up all the time, but we can offer a few guidelines for being a smart supplement shopper.

1. **You're better off sticking with a large, reputable company.** They have much more at stake than a small, unknown company. Here are some companies that enjoy strong reputations in the supplement industry: Rexall, Sundown, Thompson, Richardson Labs, and Nutramax.

2. **Don't be a bargain shopper.** There are a wide range of prices, but buying the cheapest product isn't necessarily buying smart. We suggest you look for prices in the mid to lower ranges, but don't necessarily buy the cheapest brand—as a general rule, you get what you pay for.

3. **Patents count.** Certain companies have been able to patent or license the patent to certain products. A patent is another guarantee of quality for two reasons. First, because rigorous substantiation must be presented to the patent office before a patent is issued, you can be sure there is good science behind the product. Second, the product manufacturer must ensure that the product being sold contains the exact ingredients specified in the patent. For example, in the competitive world of arthritis supplements featuring glucosamine and chondroitin, Osteo-Bi-Flex is the mass market brand authorized by the primary patent holder.

4. **Look for the warning label.** If a product makes any type of health claim, such as "promotes memory," "provides nutritional support for prostate health," or "helps maintain healthy, mobile joints and cartilage" then, by law, the manufacturer is required to run this statement: "These statements have not been evaluated by the Food and Drug Administration. This product is not intended to diagnose, treat, cure, or prevent any disease." If this wording isn't there, and the label makes a health claim, then this company is running afoul of the law and should be avoided.

5. **Check the product expiration date.** As supplements age, their potency diminishes, so keeping them around for too long is not a good idea. Remember that unless you take the product daily you may have it around for several months. Try to buy supplements with expiration dates *at least* nine months in the future.

SUGGESTED READING

BOOKS

Adderly, Brenda D. and Lissa De Angelis. *The Arthritis Cure Cookbook*. Washington, D.C.: Lifeline Press, 1998.

Adderly, Brenda D. *The Doctors' Guide to Over-the-Counter Drugs*. New York: Warner Books, 1998.

Balch, James F., and Phyllis A. Balch. *Prescription for Nutritional Healing*. Garden City Park, NY: Avery Publishing Group, 1990.

Carper, Jean. *Miracle Cures*. New York: HarperCollins, 1997.

Chevallier, Andrew. *The Encyclopedia of Medicinal Plants*. New York: DK Publishing, 1996.

Colbin, Annemarie. *Food and Healing*. New York: Ballantine, 1986.

Crook, Thomas H., Ph.D., and Brenda Adderly, M.H.A. *The Memory Cure*. New York: Pocket Books/Simon & Schuster, 1998.

Fox, Arnold, M.D., and Brenda Adderly, M.H.A. *The Fat Blocker Diet*. New York: St. Martin's Press, 1997.

Gottlieb, Bill. *New Choices in Natural Healing*. Emmaus, PA: Rodale Press, 1995.

Heinerman, John. *Heinerman's Encyclopedia of Healing Herbs & Spices*. Crystal Lake, IL: Parker Publishing, 1995.

Heinerman's Encyclopedia of Nature's Vitamins and Minerals. New Jersey: Prentice Hall, 1998.

Hendler, Sheldon Saul, M.D., Ph.D. *The Doctor's Vitamin & Mineral Encyclopedia*. New York: Simon & Schuster, 1990.

Hoffman, David. *The New Holistic Herbal.* New York: Barnes & Noble, 1983.

Kesten, Deborah. *Feeding the Body, Nourishing the Soul: Essentials of Eating for Physical, Emotional, and Spiritual Well-Being.* Berkeley, CA: Conari, 1998.

Kowalchick, Claire, and William H. Hylton, ed. *Rodale's Illustrated Encyclopedia of Herbs.* Emmaus, PA: Rodale Press, 1987.

Lieberman, Shari, Ph.D., and Nancy Burning. *The Real Vitamin & Mineral Book: Using Supplements for Optimum Health.* Garden City Park, NY: Avery Publishing Group, 1997.

McDonald, Arline, Ph.D., R.D., Annette Natow, Ph.D., R.D., Jo-Ann Heslin, M.A., R.D., Susan Male Smith, M.A., R.D. *Consumer Guide's The Complete Book of Vitamins & Minerals.* Lincolnwood, IL: Publications International, 1996.

Mindell, Earl R., Ph.D. *Earl Mindell's Food As Medicine.* New York: Fireside/Simon & Schuster, 1994. *Earl Mindell's Supplement Bible.* New York: Fireside/Simon & Schuster, 1998. *Earl Mindell's Vitamin Bible.* New York: Warner Books, 1985.

Murray, Michael T., N.D. *Encyclopedia of Nutritional Supplements.* Rocklin, CA: Prima Publishing, 1996.

Murray, Michael, N.D., and Joseph Pizzorno, N.D. *Encyclopedia of Natural Medicine.* Rocklin, CA: Prima Publishing, 1991.

Northrup, Christiane. *Women's Bodies, Women's Wisdom* 2nd ed. New York: Bantam, 1998.

Ody, Penelope. *The Complete Medicinal Herbal.* New York: DK Publishing, 1993.

Pressman, Alan, D.C., Ph.D, C.C.N., and Sheila Buff. *The Complete Idiot's Guide to Vitamins and Minerals*. New York: Alpha Books, 1997.

Preuss, Harry G., M.D., and Brenda Adderly, M.H.A. *The Prostate Cure*. New York: Crown, 1998.

Reid, Daniel. *A Handbook of Chinese Healing Herbs*. Boston: Shambahala Publications, 1995.

Ritchason, Jack. *The Vitamin and Health Encyclopedia*. Woodlands, TX: Woodland Books, 1995.

Root-Bernstein, Robert, and Michele Root-Bernstein. *Honey, Mud, Maggots, and Other Medical Marvels: The Science Behind Folk Remedies and Old Wives' Tales*. Boston: Houghton Mifflin, 1998.

Stary, Frantisek. *The Natural Guide to Medicinal Herbs and Plants*. New York: Dorset Press, 1992.

Somer, E. *Nutrition for a Healthy Pregnancy*. New York: Owl Books, 1995.

Sullivan, Karen. *The Complete Family Guide to Natural Home Remedies: Safe and Effective Treatments for Common Ailments*. New York: Barnes & Noble, 1997.

Theodosakis, Jason, M.D., M.S., M.P.H., Brenda Adderly, M.H.A., and Barry Fox, Ph.D. *The Arthritis Cure*. New York: St. Martin's Press, 1997.

Theodosakis, Jason, M.D., M.S., M.P.H., Brenda Adderly, M.H.A., and Barry Fox, Ph.D. *Maximizing the Arthritis Cure*. New York: St. Martin's Press, 1998.

Tierra, Lesley L., Ac., Herbalist. *The Herbs of Life: Health & Healing Using Western & Chinese Techniques.* Freedom, CA: Crossing Press, 1992.

Walji, Hasnain. *Health Essentials Vitamin Guide: Essential Nutrients for Healthy Living.* Rockport, MA: Element Books, 1992.

JOURNALS, NEWSPAPERS, AND MAGAZINES

Alternative Therapies
EastWest: The Journal of Natural Health & Living
The Herbal Healthline
The Herb Quarterly
The Journal of the American Medical Association (JAMA)
Lancet
Lawrence Review of Natural Products
Let's Live
Longevity
Natural Health Magazine
New England Journal of Medicine
New York Times (Jane E. Brody columns)
Nutrition
Nutrition Today
Prevention
Village Voice
The Vitamin Connection
Whole Earth Review
Whole Foods

NOTES

Acidophilus

Ayebo, A. D., I. A. Angelo, K. M. Shanahani, and C. Kies. "Effect of Feeding *Lactobacillus acidophilus* Milk Upon Fecal Flora and Enzyme Activity in Humans." *J. Dair Sci* 62 (Suppl. 1) (1979): 44–46.

Collins, M. L., and M. M. Clements. "Inhibition of *Candida albicans* by *Lactobacillus acidophilus*." *American Journal of Clinical Nutrition* 23 (1997): 713–717.

Galask, R., and B. Larsen. "Vaginal Microbial Flora: Practical and Theoretic Relevance." *OB Gyn* 55 (Suppl.) (1980): 1005–1135.

Alfalfa

Duke, John J. "Herbal Supplementation and Cholesterol?" *Atherosclerosis* 17, (June 1996): 57–71.

Aloe Vera

"Aloe Vera: The Powerful Healing Herb." *The Vitamin Connection* (November 1990): 27–29.

Fox, T. R. "Aloe Vera: Revered, Mysterious Healer." *Health Foods Business* (December 1990): 45–46.

Visuthikosol, V., et al. "Effect of Aloe Vera Gel to Healing of Burn Wound: A Clinical and Histologic Study." *J. Med Assoc. Thai* (August 1995): 67–72.

Zhou, H., and D. Jiao. "312 Cases of Gastric and Duodenal Ulcer Bleeding Treated With 3 Kinds of Alcholic Extract Rhubarb Tablets." *Chung His I Chieh Ho Tsa Shih* 10 (1990): 150–151.

Arginine

Griffith, R. D. Delong, and J. Nelson. "Relation of Arginine-Lysine Antagonism of Herpes Simplex Growth in Tissue Culture." *Chemotherapy* 27 (1981): 209–213.

Arnica

Hart, O. "Double-Blind, Placebo-Controlled, Randomized Clinical Trial of Homeopathic Arnica C30 for Pain and Infection After Total Abdominal Hysterectomy. *J.J. Soc. Med.* (February 1997).

"Nature's Medicine Cabinet." *Natural Health* (December 1996).

Astragalus

Change, H. M., and P. P. H. Buts, eds. *Pharmacology and Applications of Chinese Materia Medica*. Singapore: World Scientific, 1987.

Zhao, K. S., et al. "Enhancement of the Immune Response in Mice by Astragalus membranaceus." *Immunopharmacol* 20 (1988): 225–233.

Bilberry

Murray, M. *The Healing Power of Herbs*. Rocklin, Calif.: Prima Publishing, 1996.

Whanger, P., et al. "A Potent Natural Product for the Treatment of Rheumatoid Arthritis." *Biochemical Pharmacology* 42 (1992): 313–321.

Bioflavonoids

Ferrandiz, M. L., and J. J. Alcaraz. "Anti-Inflammatory Activity and Inhibition of Arachidonic Acid Metabolism by Flavonoids." *Agents Action* 32 (1991): 283–287.

Herzog, M. G., et al. "Dietary Antioxidant Flavonoids and Risk of Coronary Heart Disease: The Zutphen Elderly Study." *The Lancet* 342 (1993): 1007–1011.

Hirono, I., H. Ueno, S. Hosaka, et al. "Carcinogenicity Examination of Quercetin and Rutin in ACI Rats. *Cancer Letter* 13 (1981): 15–21.

Biotin
Nisenson, A. "Treatment of Seborrheic Dermatitis With Biotin and Vitamin B Complex." *Journal of Pediatrics* 81 (1972): 630–631.

Reddi, A., B. DeAngelis, O. Frank, et al. "Biotin Supplementation Improves Glucose and Insulin Tolerances in Genetically Diabetic Mice." *Life Sciences* 42 (1988): 1323–1330.

Blue-Green Algae
Romay, C. "Antioxidant and Anti-inflammatory Properties of C-phycocyanin From Blue Green Algae. *Inflamma Res.* (January 1998): 2078–2092.

"Nature's Medicine Cabinet." *Natural Health* (December 1996).

Borage
Horrobin, David F., and Mehar S. Manku. "Clinical Biochemistry of Essential Fatty Acids." *Omega-6 Essential Fatty Acids: Pathophysiology and Roles in Clinical Medicine*. New York: Alan R. Liss (1990): 21–53.

Simopoulos, A. "Omega-3 Fatty Acids in Health and Disease and in Growth and Development." *American Journal of Clinical Nutrition* (1991): 438–463.

Boron
Block, G. "Dietary Guidelines and the Results of Food Consumption Surveys." *American Journal of Clinical Nutrition* 53 (1991): 356–357.

Chapin, R. E. "The Effects of Dietary Boron on Bone Strength in Rats." *Fundamentals of Applied Toxicology* (February 1997): 161–167.

Travers, R. L., G. C. Rennie, and R. E. Newnham. "Boron and Arthritis: The Results of a Double-Blind Pilot Study." *Journal of Nutritional Medicine* 1 (1990): 127–132.

Brewer's Yeast

Glore, S. R., et al. "Soluble Fiber and Serum Lipids: A Literature Review." *Journal of the American Dietary Association* 94 (1994): 425–436.

Bromelain

Rimoldi, R., F. Ginesu, and R. Giura. "The Use of Bromelain in Pneumolical Therapy," *Drugs Exp Clin* 4 (1978): 55–66.

Ryan, R. "A Double-Blind Clinical Evaluation of Bromelains in the Treatment of Acute Sinusitis." *Headache* 7 (1967): 13–17.

Calcium

Block, G. "Dietary Guidelines and the Results of Food Consumption Surveys." *American Journal of Clinical Nutrition* 53 (1991): 356–357.

Licata, A. et al. "Acute Effects of Dietary Protein on Calcium Metabolism in Patients With Osteoporosis." *Journal of Gerontology* 36 (1981): 14–19.

Zhou, C., et al. "Clinical Observation of Treatment of Hypertension With Calcium." *American Journal of Hypertension* 7 (1994): 363–367.

Carnitine

Kanter, M. M., et al. "Antioxidants, Carnitine, and Choline as Putative Erogegenic Aids." *International Journal of Sports Nutrition* (1995): 120–131.

Cat's Claw

Hipepo, J. N. "Acute Renal Failure Caused by 'Cat's Claw' Herbal Remedy in a Patient With Systemic Lupus (Letter)." *Nephron* (1997).

"Nature's Medicine Cabinet." *Natural Health* (December 1996).

Cayenne Pepper

Castleman, M. "Red Pepper Is Hot." *Medical Selfcare* (September–October 1989).

Ellis, C. N., et al. "A Double-Blind Evaluation of Topical Capsaicin in Pruritic Psoriasis." *Journal American Academy of Dermatology* 29 (1993): 438–442.

Cernitin

Becker, H., and L. Ebeling. "Conservative Treatment of Benign Prostatic Hyperplasia (BPH) With Cernilton N." *Urologe* (B) 28 (1988): 301–306.

Preuss, H., and B. Adderly. *The Prostate Cure.* New York: Crown, 1998.

Rugendorff, E. W., W. Weidner, L. Ebeling, and A. C. Buck. "Results of Treatment With Pollen Extract (Cernilton N) in Chronic Prostatitis and Prostadynia." *British Journal of Urology* 71 (1993): 433–438.

Chamomile

Mann, B., and E. J. Staba. "The Chemistry, Pharmacology, and Commercial Formulations of Chamomile." *Herbs, Spices, and Medicinal Plants* 1 (1984): 235–280.

Yamada, K. "Effect of Inhalation of Chamomile Oil Vapour on Plasma ACTH Level in Ovariectomized Rat Under Restriction Stress." *Biol Pharm Bull* (September 1996): 274–277.

Chitosan

Deuchi, K., et al. "Decreasing Effect of Chitosan on the Apparent Fat Digestibility by Rats Fed on a High-Fat Diet." *Bioscience Biotechnology Biochemistry* (1994): 58, 1613–1616.

Fox, A., and B. Adderly. *The Fat Blocker Diet*. New York: St Martin's Press, 1997.

Nauss, J. L., J. J. Thompson, and J. Nagyvary. "The Binding of Micellar Lipids to Chitosan." (1995) *Lipids* 18 (10): 714–719.

Yuji, M., et al. "Hypocholesterolemic Effect of Chitosan in Adult Males." *Bioscience Biotechnology Biochemistry* (May 1995): 786–790.

Chlorophyll

Ferrandiz, M. L., and J. J. Alcaraz. "Anti-Inflammatory Activity and Inhibition of Arachidonic Acid Metabolism by Flavonoids. *Agents Action* 32 (1991): 283–287.

Negishi, T. "Antigenotoxic Activity of Natural Chlorophylls." *Mutat Res.* (May 12, 1997): 1101-1110.

Sakar. D. "Clastogenic Activity of Pure Chlorophyll and Anticlastogenic Effects of Equivalent Amounts of Crude Extract of Indian Spinach Leaf and Chlorophyllin Following Dietary Supplementation to Mice." *Environ Mol Mutagen* 32 (1996): 55-67.

Choline

Kanter, M. M., et al. "Antioxidants, Carnitine, and Choline as Putative Erogegenic Aids." *International Journal of Sports Nutrition* (1995): 120–131.

Schenker, S., et al. "Polyunsaturated Lethicin and Alcoholic Liver Disease: A Magic Bulllet?" *Alcoholism: Clin. Exp. Res.* (1994): 1286–1288.

Chondroitin and Glucosamine

Crolle, G., and E. D'Este. "Glucosamine Sulphate for the Management of Arthrosis: a Controlled Clinical Investigation." *Current Medical Research and Opinion* (1980) 7 (2): 104–109.

Dovanti, A., A. A. Bignamini, and A. L. Rovati "Therapeutic Activity of Oral Glucosamine Sulphate in Osterarthritis: A Placebo-Controlled Double-Blind Investigation." *Clinical Therapeutics* (1980) 3 (4): 266–272.

Mazi'res, B., et al. "Le chondroitin sulfate dans le traitement de la gonarthrose et de al coxarthrose." *Rev Rheum Mal Ostéoartic* (1992) 59 (7–8): 466–472.

Pipitone, V. R., "Chondroprotection with Chondroitin Sulfate." *Drugs in Experimental and Clinical Research* (1991) 17 (1): 3–7.

Theodosakis, J., B. Adderly, and B. Fox. *The Arthritis Cure.* New York: St. Martin's Press, 1997.

Theodosakis, J., B. Adderly, and B. Fox. *Maximizing the Arthritis Cure.* New York: St. Martin's Press, 1998.

Chromium

Anderson, R. A. "Chromium, Glucose Tolerance and Diabetes," *Biological Trace Element Research* 32 (1992): 661–667.

Press, R.J., et al. "The Effect of Chromium Piccolinate on Serum Cholesterol and Apolipoprotein Fractions on Human Subjects." *The Western Journal of Medicine* (January 1990): 29–30.

Cod Liver Oil

Horrobin, David F., and Mehar S. Manku. "Clinical Biochemistry of Essential Fatty Acids." *In Omega-6 Essential Fatty Acids: Pathophysiology and Roles in Clinical Medicine.* New York: Alan R. Liss, 1990.

Simpopoulos, A. "Omega-3 Fatty Acids in Health and Disease and in Growth and Development." *American Journal of Clinical Nutrition* (1991): 438–463.

Coenzyyme Q 10
Baggio, E., et al. "Italian Multicenter Study on the Safety and Efficacy of Co20 Therapy in Patients With Congestive Heart Failure. Co20 Drug Surveillance Investigators." *Mol Aspects Med* 15 (1994): 287–294.

Kamikawa, T., et al. "Effects of Coenzyme Q10 on Exercise Tolerance in Chronic Stable Angina Pectoris." *American Journal of Cardiology* (1985): 247–251.

Langsjoen, H., et al. "Usefulness of CoQ10 in Clinical Cardiology: A Long-term Study." *Mol Aspects Med* 15 (1994): 165–175.

Copper
Klevay, L. M., "Dietary Copper: A Powerful Determinant off Cholesterolemia." *Medical Hypotheses* 24 (1987): 111–119.

Solomons, N. W., "Biochemical, Metabolic, and Clinical Role of Copper in Human Nutrition." *J Am Coll Nutr* 4 (1985): 83-105.

Walker, W. R., and D. M. Keas. "An Investigation of the Therapeutic Value of the 'Copper Bracelet'—Dermal Assimilation of Copper in Arthritic/Rheumatoid Conditions." *Agents and Actions* 6 (1976): 454–458.

Cranberry
Kahn, D. H., et al. "Effect of Cranberry Juice on the Urine." *Journal of the American Dietetic Association* 51 (1967): 251.

Sobota, A. E. "Inhibition of Bacterial Adherence by Cranberry Juice: Potential Use for the Treatment of Urinary Tract Infections." *Journal of Urology* 131 (1984): 1013–1016.

Creatine
C. P. Earnest "The Effect of Creatine Monohydrate Ingestion on Anaerobic Power Indices, Muscular Strength and Body Composition." *Acta Physiol. Scand.* (1995): 207–209.

Cysteine
Schneider, E. L., and J. D. Reed "Life Extension." *The New England Journal of Medicine* 312 (1985): 1159–1168.

Dandelion
Williams, C. A. "Flavonoids, Cinnamic Acids, and Coumarins From the Different Tissues and Medicinal Preparations of *Taraxacum officinale*." *Phytochemistry* (May 1996): 47–61.

Murray, M. *The Healing Power of Herbs* Rocklin, Calif.: Prima Publishing, 1996.

Devil's Claw
Brady, L. R., V. E. Tyler, and J. E. Robbers. *Pharmacognosy*, 8th ed., Philadelphia: Lea & Febiger, 1981.

Whitehouse, L. W., M. Znamirowski, and C. J. Paul. "Devil's Claw: Evidence for Anti-Inflammatory Activity in the Treatment of Arthritic Disease." *Canadian Medical Association Journal* 129 (1983): 249–251.

DHEA
Morales, J., et al. "Effect of Replacement Dose of DHEA in Men and Women of Advancing Age." *Journal of Clinical Endocrinology Metabolism* (1994): 1360–1367.

Schneider, L., and J. D. Reed. "Life Extension." *The New England Journal of Medicine* 312 (1985): 1159–1168.

Dong Quai

Harada, M., M. Suzuki, and Y. Ozaki. "Effect of Japanese Angelica Root and Peony Root on Uterine Contraction in the Rabbit in Situ." *J Pharm Dyn* 7 (1984): 304–311.

Echinacea

Bauer, R., and H. Wagner. "Echinacea Species as Potential Immuno-stimulatory Drugs." *Econ Med Plant Res* 5 (1991): 253–321.

Erhard, M., et al. "Effect of Echinacea, Aconitum, Lachesis, and Apis Extracts and Their Combinations on Phagocytosis of Human Granulocytes." *Phytother Res* 8 (1994): 14–17.

Elderberry

Mumcuoglu, M., et al. "Inhibition of Several Strains of Influenza Virus in Vitro and Reduction of Symptoms by an Elderberry Extract." *The Journal of Alternative and Complementary Medicine* (1995): 361–369.

Electrolytes

Fleiss, Paul, M.D. "Quick and Simple First Aid for Your Kids." *Mothering* (August 1996): 44–49.

Oli, M. V. "Evaluation of Fructooligosaccharide Supplementation of Oral Electrolyte Solutions for Treatment of Diarrhea; Recovery of the Intestinal Bacteria." *Dig Dis Sci.* (January 1998): 14411–1417.

Peters, H. P. "Gastrointestinal Symptoms During Exercise: The Effect of Fluid Supplementation." *Sports Medicine* (August 1995): 34–37.

Eucalyptus

Pattnaik, S. "Antibacterial and Antifungal Activity of Ten Essential Oils in Vitro." *Microbios* 12 (August 1996): 981–988.

Riechelmann, H. "Response of Human Cilated Respiratory Cells to a Mixture of Menthol, Eucalyptus Oil, and Pine Needle Oil." *Arzheimittelforschung* (September 1997): 131–142.

Evening Primrose

Briggs, C. J. "Evening Primrose: La Belle de Nuit, The King's Cure-all." *Canadian Pharmacy Journal* (1987) 119 (5): 249–252, 254.

Hasssam, A. G. "The Role of Evening Primrose Oil in Nutrition and Disease." *In the Role of Fats in Human Nutrition.* Chichester, England: Ellis Horwood, 1985.

"Oil of Evening Primrose." *Lawrence Review of Natural Products* (March 1989): 22–24.

Simopoulos, A. "Omega-3 Fatty Acids in Health and Disease and in Growth and Development." *American Journal of Clinial Nutrition* (1991): 438–463.

Fennel

Jensen-Jarolim, E. "Characterization of Allergens in Apiaceae Spices: Anice, Fennel, Coriander, and Cumin." *Clinical Exp. Allergy* (November 1997): 222–233.

Fenugreek

Bordia, A. "Effect of Ginger and Fenugreek on Blood Lipids' Blood Sugar and Platelet Aggregation in Patients With Coronary Artery Disease." *Prostaglandins Leukot Essent Fatty Acids* (May 1997): 13–19.

Sharma, R. D., et al. "Effect of Fenugreek Seeds on Blood Glucose and Serum Lipids in Type I Diabetes." *Eur J. Clin Nutr* 44 (1990): 301–306.

Mada, J., et al. "Glucose-Lowering Effect of Fenugreek in Non-Insulin-Dependent Diabetics." *Eur J. Clin Nutr* 42 (1988): 51–54.

Feverfew

Johnson, E. S. *Feverfew: A Traditional Herbal Remedy for Migraine and Arthritis.* London: Sheldon Press, 1984.

Johnson, E. S., N. P. Kadam, D. M. Hylands, and P. J. Hylands. "Efficacy of Feverfew as Prohpylactic Treatment of Migraine." *British Medical Journal* (August 31, 1985) 291 (6495): 569–573.

Murphy, J. J., S. Heptinstall, and J. R. A. Mitchell. "Randomized Double-Blind Placebo Controlled Trial of Feverfew in Migraine Prevention." *Lancet* (July 23, 1988): 189–192.

Flaxseed Oil

Flax Facts." *Journal of the National Cancer Institute* (September 7, 1991) 83 (15): 1050–1052.

Horrobin, David F., and Mehar S. Manku. "Clinical biochemistry of Essential Fatty Acids." *Omega-6 Essential Fatty Acids: Pathophysiology and Roles in Clinical Medicine.* New York: Alan R. Liss, 1990: 21–53.

Simopoulos, A., "Omega-3 Fatty Acids in Health and Disease and in Growth and Development." *American Journal of Clinial Nutrition* (1991): 438–463.

Folate

Block, G. "Dietary Guidelines and the Results of Food Consumption Surveys." *American Journal of Clinical Nutrition* 53 (1991): 356–357.

Joosten, E., et al. "Metabolic Evidence That Deficiencies of Vitamin B_6 and Folate Occur Commonly in Older People." American Journal of Clinical Nutrition (1993): 468–476.

Krause, M. V., and L. K. Mahan. *Food, Nutrition, and Diet Therapy,* 5th ed. Philadelphia: WB Saunders, 1984.

Garlic

Agarwal, K. C. "Therapeutic Action of Garlic Constituents." *Med Res Rev* 16 (January 1996): 111–124.

Berthold, H., et al "A Study Indicating That Garlic Does Not Lower Serum Cholesterol." *Journal of the American Medical Association* (June 1998): 2217–2232.

Hung, O. L., et al. "Herbal Preparation Use Among Urban Emergency Department Patients." *Academy of Emergency Medicine* 31 (March 1997): 171–173.

Krause, M.V., and L. K. Mahan. *Food, Nutrition, and Diet Therapy,* 5th ed. Philadelphia: WB Saunders, 1984.

Markam, A., et al. "The Garlic Miracle." *American Journal of Clinical Nutrition* (1997): 321–323.

Stolzenburg, W. "Garlic Medicine: Cure in Cloves?" *Science News* (September 8, 1990): 74–79.

Geranium

Pattnaik, S. "Antibacterial and Antifungal Activity of Ten Essential Oils in Vitro." *Microbios* 42 (August 1996): 479–485.

SerkedJieva, J. "Inhibition of Influenza Virus Protein Synthesis by a Plant Preparation From Geranium." *Acta Virol* (February 1995): 17–19.

Ginger

Arfeen, Z. "A Double-Blind Randomized Controlled Trial of Ginger for the Prevention of Postoperative Nausea and Vomiting." *Anesthesia Intensive Care* 12 (August 1995): 71–75.

Bordia, A. "Effect of Ginger and Fenugreek on Blood Lipids' Blood Sugar and Platelet Aggregation in Patients With Coronary Artery

Disease." *Prostaglandins Leukot Essent Fatty Acids* (May 1997): 299–307.

Fischer-Rasmussen, W., et al. "Ginger Treatment of Hyperemesis Gravidarum." *Eur J. Obstet Gynecoll Reprod Biol* 38 (1990): 19–24.

Hung, O.L., et al. "Herbal Preparation Use Among Urban Emergency Department Patients." *Academy of Emergency Medicine* (March 1997): 617–624.

Phillips, S. "*Zingiber officinale* (ginger—an Antiemetic for Day Case Surgery." *Anaesthesia* 17 (August 1993): 131–139.

Gingko
Chen, X. "Progress of Pharmacological Research on Cardiovascular and Cerebrovascular Effects of Gingko Biloba Extracts and Its Enlightenment." *Chung Kuo Chung His I Chieh Ho Tsa Chih* (July 1996): 3217–3231.

Herve, A., et al. "Effect of Two Doses of Gingko Biloba Extract on the Dual-Coding Test in Elderly Subjects" *Clinical Therapeutics,* 549–558.

Kleijnin, J., et al. "Gingko Biloba." *Lancet* (1992): 1136–1139.

LeBars, P. L., et al. "A Placebo-Controlled, Double-Blind, Randomized Trial of an Extract of Ginkgo Biloba for Dementia." *Journal of the American Medical Association* 278 (1997): 1327–1332.

"Minding Your Memory With Ginkgo?" *The Johns Hopkins Medical Letter* (February 1998).

Ginseng
Choi, H. K., "Clinical Efficacy of Korean Red Ginseng for Erectile Dysfunction." *Int J. Impot Res* (September 1995): 12–17.

Wagner, H., et al. "Siberian Ginseng: Current Status as an Adaptogen." In *Economic and Medicinal Plant Research*. London: Academic Press, 1995.

Yun, T. K. "Preventative Effect of Ginseng Intake Against Various Human Cancers: a Case-Control Study on 1987 Pairs." *Cancer Epidemiol Biomarkers Prev* (June 1995): 849–857.

Glutamine & Glutamic Acid

Yoo, S. S. "Glutamine Supplementation Maintains Intramuscular Glutamine Concentrations and Normalizes Digestive Function in Early Weaned Pigs." *Journal of Nutrition* (November 1997).

Ziegler, T. R. "Glutamine Supplementation in Catabolic Illness." *American Journal of Clinical Nutrition* (October 1996): 1377–1382.

Goldenseal

Hung, O. L., et al. "Herbal Preparation Use Among Urban Emergency Department Patients." *Academy of Emergency Medicine* (March 1997): 485-491.

Kumazawa, Y., et al. "Activation of Peritoneal Macrophages by Be Terms of Induction of Cytostatic Activity." *Int J Immunopharmacol* 6 (1984): 387–394.

Gotu Kola

Boiteau, P., and A. R. Ratsimamanga. "Asiaticoside Extracted From *Centella Asiatica*, Its Therapeutic Uses in the Healing of Experimental or Refractory Wounds, Leprosy, Skin Tuberculosis, and Lupus." *Therapie* (1992) 11: 125–149.

Bolgert, M., and G. Gautron. "An Extract Form *Centella asiatica* in Phlebology." *Prog Med* (France) 100 (1972): 31–32.

Green-Lipped Mussel Extract

DeWith, N. D. "Intracellular Degradation of C-Peptides in Molluscan Neurons Producing Insulin-Related Hormones." *Peptides* (1997): 32–39.

Jung, S. "Are Glycosaminogluycans Responsible for the Therapeutic Effect of Mussel Extract? A Contribution to the Current Controversy." *Tierarztl Prax Ausg K. Klientiere Heimtiere* (February 1998): 7–10.

Murray, M., and J. Pizzorno. *Encylopedia of Natural Medicine.* 2nd ed. Rocklin, Calif.: Prima Publishing, 1996.

Hawthorn

Bahorun, T. "Oxygen Species Scavenging Activity of Phenolic Extracts From Hawthorn Fresh Plant Organs and Pharmaceutical Preparations." *Arzheimittelforschung* (November 1996): 222–231.

Popping, S. "Effect of a Hawthorn Extract on Contraction and Energy Turnover of Isolated Rat Cardiomyocytes." *Arzheimittelforschung* (November 1995): 112–117.

Iodine

Block, G. "Dietary Guidelines and the Results of Food Consumption Surveys." *American Journal of Clinical Nutrition* 53 (1991): 171-174.

Furudate, S. "1251 Uptake Competing With Iodine Absorption by the Thyroid Gland Following Povidone-Iodine Skin Application." *Exp Anim* (July 1997).

Kalk, W. J. "Thyroid Cancer in South Africa—an Indicator of Regional Iodine Deficiency." *S. African Medical Journal* (June 1997): 398–411.

Iron

Block, G. "Dietary Guidelines and the Results of Food Consumption Surveys." *American Journal of Clinical Nutrition* 53 (1991): 382–395.

Juniper

Pattnaik, S. "Antibacterial and Antifungal Activity of Ten Essential Oils in Vitro." *Microbios* (August 1996): 1271–1279.

Schilcher, H. "Juniper Berry Oil in Diseases of the Urinary Tract." *Med Monatsschr Pharm.* (July 1995): 813–819.

"The Potential Nephrotoxic Effects of Essential Juniper Oil." *Arzneimittelforschung* (July 1997): 298–307.

Kava

Singh, Y. N. "Kava: An Overview." *Journal of Ethnopharmacology* (1996): 13–45.

Volz, H. P. "Kava-Kava Extract WS 1490 Versus Placebo in Anxiety Disorders—a Randomized Placebo-Controlled 25-Week Outpatient Trial." *Pharmacopsychiatry* (January 1997): 788–792.

Kelp/Bladderwrack

Block, G. "Dietary Guidelines and the Results of Food Consumption Surveys." *American Journal of Clinical Nutrition* 53 (1991): 356–357.

Kombucha Mushroom

Srinivasan, R., S. Smolinski, and D. Greenbaum. "Probable Gastrointestinal Toxicity of Kombucha Tea: Is This Beverage Healthy or Harmful?" *Journal of General Internal Medicine* 12 (October 1997): 643–644.

Lady's Mantle

Siegal, H. "Nutriceutical Review of Lady's Mantle (*Alchemilla vulgaris*) for the Treatment of Premenstrual Syndrome (PMS)." *Journal of Women's Health,* (August 1995): 198–208.

"Nature's Medicine Cabinet." *Natural Health* (December 1996).

Lavender

Cornwell, S. "Lavender Oil and Perineal Repair." *Modern Midwife* (March 1995): 37–42.

Pattnaik, S. "Antibacterial and Antifungal Activity of Ten Essential Oils in Vitro." *Microbios* (August 1996): 109–117.

Lecithin

Schenker, A., et al. "Polyunsaturated Lethicin and Alcoholic Liver Disease: A Magic Bullet?" *Alcoholism: Clin Exp Res* (1994): 1286–1288.

Licorice

Armanini, D. "Further Studies on the Mechanism of the Mineralocorthicoid Action of Licorice in Humans." *J. Endocrinol Invest* (October 1996): 67–72.

Vaya, J. "Antioxidant Constituents From Licorice Roots: Isolation, Structure Elucidation, and Antioxidative Capacity Toward LDL Oxidation." *Free Radic Biol Med* (1997): 1347–1351.

Lysine

Flodin, N. W., et al. "The Metabolic Roles, Pharmacology and Toxicity of Lysine." *American Journal of Clinical Nutrition* 16 (1) 7–21 (1997).

Griffith, R., D. DeLong, and J. Nelson. "Relation of Arginine-Lysine Antagonism of Herpes Simplex Growth in Tissue Culture." *Chemotherapy* 27 (1981): 209–213.

Magnesium

Altura, B., et al. "Magnesium: Growing in Clinical Importance." *Patient Care* (January 15, 1994): 130–131.

Ma Huang

Theoharides, T. C. "Sudden Death of a Healthy College Student Related to Ephedrine Toxicity From a Ma Huang-Containing Drink." *Journal of Clinical Psychopharmacology* 37 (October 1997): 917–922.

White, L. M. "Pharmacokinetics and Cardiovascular Effects of Ma Huang in Normotensive Adults." *Journal of Clinical Pharmacology* (February 1997).

Manganese

Keen, C. L. and S. Zidenberg-Cherr. *Manganese: Present Knowledge in Nutrition*, 6th ed. Washington, D.C.: International Life Sciences Institute, 1990.

Melatonin

Bahorun, T. "A Review of the Evidence Supporting Melatonin's Role as an Antioxidant," *Arzheimittelforschung* (November 1997): 317–323.

Pierpaoli, W., et al. *The Melatonin Miracle*. New York: Simon & Schuster, 1995.

Methionine & Taurrine

Krause, M. V. and L. K. Mahan. *Food, Nutrition, and Diet Therapy*, 5th ed. Philadelphia: WB Saunders, 1984.

Zaman, N. "Effects of Taurine Supplementation in Parenteral Nutrition-Associated Hepatosteatosis and Lidocaine Metabolism." *Drug Metab Dispos* (May 1996): 788794.

Milk Thistle
Von Schonfeld, J. "Silbinin, a Plant Extract With Antioxidant and Membrane Stabilizing Properties, Protects Exocrine Pancreas From Cyclosporin A Toxcity." *Lehrbuch der Phytotherapie* (December 1997): 112–115.

Molybdenum
Sardesai, V. M. "Molybdenum: An Essential Trace Element. *Nutr Clin Prac* 8 (1993): 277–281.

Motherwort
Harada, M., M. Suzuki, and Y. Ozaki, "Effect of Japanese Angelica Root and Peony Root on Uterine Contraction in the Rabbit in Situ," *J Pharm Dyn* 7 (1984): 304–311.

Niacin (Vitamin B₃)
Block, G. "Dietary Guidelines and the Results of Food Consumption Surveys." *American Journal of Clinical Nutrition* 53 (1991): 356–357.

Krause, M. V., and L. K. Mahan. *Food, Nutrition, and Diet Therapy,* 5th ed. Philadelphia: WB Saunders, 1984.

PABA
Allen, J. M. "Photochemical Formation of Singlet Molecular Oxygen in Illuminated Aqueous Solutions of Several Commercially Available Sunscreen Active Ingredients." *Chem Res Toxicol* (April–May 1996).

Tanojo, H. "In Vitro Human Skin Barrier Modulation by Fatty Acids: Skin Permeation and Thermal Analysis Studies." *Pharm Res* (January 1997): 161–166.

Pau d'arco

Dinnen, R. D. "The Search for Novel Anticancer Agents: A Differentiation-Based Assay and Analysis of a Folklore Product." *Anticancer Research* 22 (March-April, 1997): 153–164.

Peony

Harada, M., M. Suzuki, and Y. Ozaki. "Effect of Japanese Angelica Root and Peony Root on Uterine Contraction in the Rabbit in Situ," *J Pharm Dyn* 7 (1984): 304-311.

Peppermint

Beesley, A. "Influence on Peppermint Oil on Absorptive and Secretory Process in Small Rat Intestine." *Gut* (August 1996).

Mindell, E. *Earl Mindell's Herb Bible.* New York: Fireside, 1992.

Pattnaik S. "Antibacterial and Antifungal Activity of Ten Essential Oils in Vitro." *Microbios* (August 1996): 279–284.

Phenylalanine

Hyland K. "Oral Phenylalanine Loading in Dopa-Responsive Dystonia: A Possible Diagnostic Test." *Neurology* (May 1997): 343-351.

Nakamura, K. "Quantitation of L-amino Acids by Substrate Recycling Between an Aminotransferase and a Dehydrogenase: Application to the Determination of L-phenylalanine in Human Blood." *Anal Biochemistry* 22 (February 1, 1996): 15-19.

Phosphatidylserine (PS)

Cenacchi, T., et al. "Cognitive Decline in the Elderly: A Double-Blind, Placebo-Controlled Multicenter Study on Efficacy of Phosphatidylserine Administration." *Aging (Milano)* (April 1993) 5 (2): 123–133.

Crook, T., and B. Adderly. *The Memory Cure.* New York: Pocket Books, 1998.

Crook, T. H., et al. "Effects of Phosphatidylserine in Age Associated Memory Impairmant." *Neurology* 41 (May 1991): 644–649.

Phosphorous
Krause, M. V., and L. K. Mahan. *Food, Nutrition, and Diet Therapy,* 5th ed. Philadelphia: WB Saunders, 1984.

Murray, M., and J. Pizzorno. *Enclyclopedia of Natural Medicine,* 2nd ed. Rocklin, Calif.: Prima Publishing, 1996.

Psyllium
Bailey, Steven. *Passage 23.* Portland, Ore.: Northwest Naturopathic Clinic, 1998.

Glore, S. R., et al. "Soluble Fiber and Serum Lipids: A Literature Review." *Journal of the American Dietary Association* 94 (1994): 425–436.

Rosemary
Kumura, Y. "German Study on the Effects of Rosemary on the Brain." *Arnheim Ass* (March 1996).

Pattnaik, S. "Antibacterial and Antifungal Activity of Ten Essential Oils in Vitro." *Microbios* 13 (August 1996): 971–998.

Royal Jelly
Leung, R. "Royal Jelly Consumption and Hypersensitivity in the Community." *Clin Exp Allergy* (March 1997): 172–177.

Thien, F. C. "Asthma and Anaphylaxix Induced by Royal Jelly." *Clin Exp Allergy* 29 (February 1996): 414–421.

Saw Palmetto

Braeckman, J. "The Extract of Serenoa Repens in the Treatment of Benign Prostatic Hyperplasia: A Multi-Center Open Study." *Current Therapeutic Research, Clinical and Experimental* 55 (1994): 776–785.

Champault, G., et al. "A Double-Blind Trial of an Extract of the Plant Serenoa Repens in Benign Prostatic Hyperplasia." *British Journal of Clinical Pharmacology* (1984) 18, 461–462.

Selenium

Fan, A. M., and K. W. Kizer. "Selenium: Nutritional, Toxilogical, and Clinical Aspects." *West J. Med* 153 (1990): 160–167.

Mutanen, M. "Bioavailability of Selenium." *Annals Clin Res* 18 (1986): 48–54.

Shark Cartilage

Kail, K. "Use of Shark Cartilage to Inhibit Angiogenesis." *New England Journal of Medicine* (July 1985): 488–499.

Slippery Elm

Mindell, E. *Earl Mindell's Herb Bible*. New York: Fireside, 1992.

Murray, M., and J. Pizzorno. *Encyclopedia of Natural Medicine*, 2nd ed. Rocklin, Calif.: Prima Publishing, 1996.

Soy

Barnes, S., et al., "Soybeans Inhibit Mammary Tumors in Models of Breast Cancer." *Mutagens and Carcinogens in Diet* (1990): 145–149.

Messina, M., et al. "Soy Intake and Cancer Risk: A Review of the In Vitro and In Vivo Data." *Nutrition and Cancer* (1994): 12–17.

St. John's Wort

Bloomfield, Harold. *Hypericum and Depression.* New York: Prelude Press, 1997.

"Can You Tell Me About St. John's Wort? I've Been Depressed and Wonder If It Would Be Safe to Take." *Mayo Clinic Health Letter* (May 1998).

Lieberman, S. "Nutriceutical Review of St. John's Wort (*Hypericum perforatum*) for the Treatment of Depression." *Journal of Women's Health* (March 1998).

Miller, A. L. "St. John's Wort (*Hypericum perforatum*): Clinical Effects on Depression and Other Conditions." *Alternative Medicine Review* (February 1998): 778–787.

Tea

Gao, Y. T., et al. "Reduced Risk of Esophageal Cancer Associated With Green Tea Consumption." *Journal of the National Cancer Institute* (June 1, 1994): 855–858.

Katiyar, S. K., R. Agarwal, and H. Mukhtar. "Green Tea in Chemoprevention of Cancer." *Compr, Ther,* 18 (1992): 3–8.

Yang, C. S., and Z. Y. Wang. "Tea and Cancer." *Journal of the National Cancer Institute* 85 (1993): 1038–1049.

Tryptophan

Birlouez-Aragon, I. "Effect of Iron and Lactose Supplementation of Milk on the Maillard Reaction and Tryptophan Content." *Food Additive Contamination* (May-June 1997): 306–311.

Krause, M. V. and L. K. Mahan. *Food, Nutrition, and Diet Therapy,* 5th ed. Philadelphia: WB Saunders, 1984.

Tyrosine
Krause, M. V., and L. K. Mahan. *Food, Nutrition, and Diet Therapy,* 5th ed. Philadelphia: WB Saunders, 1984.

Rohr, F. J. "Tyrosine Supplementation in the Treatment of Maternal Phenylketonuria." *American Journal of Clinical Nutrition* 48 (March 1998): 2827–2832.

Valerian
Gerhard, U. "Vigilance-Decreasing Effects of 2 Plant-Derived Sedatives." *Schweiz Rundsch Med Prax* (April 9, 1996): 381–388.

Oshima, Y. "Antidepressant Principles of Valerianan Fauriei Roots." *Chem Pharm Bull.* Tokyo, January 1995.

Vitamin A
Block, G. "Dietary Guidelines and the Results of Food Consumption Surveys." *American Journal of Clinical Nutrition* 53 (1991): 356–357.

Krause, M. V., and L. K. Mahan. *Food, Nutrition, and Diet Therapy,* 5th ed. Philadelphia: WB Saunders, 1984.

Mangels, A. R., et al. "Carotenoid Content of Fruits and Vegetables: An Evaluation of Analytic Data." *Journal of the American Dietetic Association* 93 (1993): 284–286.

Seddon, J., et al. "Dietary Carotenoids, Viatmins A, C, and E, and Advanced Age-Related Macular Degeneration." *Journal of the American Medical Association* 18 (1994): 1413–1420.

Vitamin B_1
Block, G. "Dietary Guidelines and the Results of Food Consumption Surveys." *American Journal of Clinical Nutrition* 53 (1991): 356–357.

Krause, M. V., and L. K. Mahan. *Food Nutrition, and Diet Therapy,* 5th ed. Philadelphia: WB Saunders, 1984.

Vitamin B$_2$

Block, G. "Dietary Guidelines and the Results of Food Consumption Surveys." *American Journal of Clinical Nutrition* 53 (1991): 356–357.

Vitamin B$_5$

Cigetti, G., et al. "Effects of Pantethine on Cholesterol Synthesis from Mevalonate Is Isolated Rate Hepatocytes." *Atherosclerosos* (1986) 60 (1): 67-77.

Fry P.C., et al. "Metabolic Response to a Pantothenic Acid Deficient Diet in Humans." *J. Nutr Sci Vitaminol* 22 (1976): 339-346.

Vitamin B$_6$ (Pyridoxine)

Block, G. "Dietary Guidelines and the Results of Food Consumption Surveys." *American Journal of Clinical Nutrition* 53 (1991): 356–357.

Joosten, E., et al. "Metabolic Evidence That Deficiencies of Vitamin B$_6$ and Folate Occur Commonly in Older People." *American Journal of Clinical Nutrition* 36 (1993): 468-476.

Rall, L., et al. "Vitamin B$_6$ and Immune Competence." *Nutrition Reviews* (1993): 217-225.

Vitamin C

Block, G. "Dietary Guidelines and the Results of Food Consumption Surveys." *American Journal of Clinical Nutrition* 53 (1991): 356–357.

Pauling, L. *Vitamin C and the Common Cold.* San Francisco: Freeman, 1970.

Pinnel, S., et al. "Induction of Collagen Synthesis by Ascorbic Acid: A Possible Mechanism." *Archives of Dermatology* (1987): 1684–1686.

Seddon, J., et al. "Dietary Carotenoids, Vitamins A, C, and E, and Advanced Age-Related Macular Degeneration," *Journal of the American Medical Association* 18 (1994): 1413–1420.

Vitamin D
Garland, C. F., and F. C. Garland. "Do Sunlight and Vitamin D Reduce the Likelihood of Cancer?" *Int J. Epidemiol* 9 (1980): 227–231.

Gloth, F. M., and H. D. Tobin. "Vitamin D Deficiency in Older People." *J Am Geriatr Soc* 43 (1995): 822–828.

Lore, F., et al. "Vitamin D Metabolites in Postmenopausal Osteoporosis." *Horm Metabol Res* 16 (1984): 58–61.

Vitamin E
Bellizzi, M. C. et al. "Vitamin E and Coronary Heart Disease: The European Paradox." *Eur J Clin Nutr* 48 (1994): 822–831.

Stevens, N. G., et al. "Randomized Controlled Trial of Vitamin E in Patients With Coronary Disease: Cambridge Heart Antioxidant Study." *Lancet* (March 23, 1996): 781-786.

Seddon, J., et al. "Dietary Carotenoids, Vitamins A, C, and E, and Advanced Age-Related Macular Degeneration," *Journal of the American Medical Association* 18 (1994): 1413–1420.

Vitamin K
Suttie, J. W. "Vitamin K and Human Nutrition." *J Am Diet Assoc* 92 (1993): 585–590.

Wild Yam

Lee, J. R. "Osteoporosis Reversal: The Role of Progesterone." *International Clinical Nutrition Review* (1990): 384–391.

Prior, J. C. "Progesterone as a Bone-Tropic Hormone." *Endocrine Reviews* (1990): 386–398.

Witch Hazel

Fleiss, Paul, M.D. "Quick and Simple First Aid for Your Kids." *Mothering,* (August, 1996): 44–49.

Murray, M., and J. Pizzorno. *Encyclopedia of Natural Medicine.* 2nd ed. Rocklin, Calif.: Prima Publishing, 1996.

Woolwine, J. D. "Effect of Testing Method on Apparent Activities of Antiviral Disinfectants and Antiseptics." *Antimicrob Agents Chemother* (April 1995): 7–11.

Yucca

Mindell, E. *Earl Mindell's Herb Bible.* New York: Fireside, 1992.

Shull, M.A., et.al. "Saponin Supplementation Successfully Relieves Osteoarthritis Symptoms." *The Journal of Applied Nutrition* 17 (1993): 258–262.

Zinc

Eby, G. A., D. R. Davis, and W. W. Halcomb. "Reduction in Duration of Common Colds by Zinc Gluconate Lozenges in a Double-Blind Study." *Antimicrob Agents Chemoter* 5 (1994): 20–25.

Macknin, M. L., M. Piedmonte, et al. "Zinc Gluconate Lozenges for Treating the Common Cold in Children; a Randomized Controlled Trial." *Journal of the American Medical Association* (June 24, 1998) 279 (24): 1962–1967.

INDEX

Dear Reader:

Thank you for buying *The Complete Guide to Nutritional Supplements*. My specialty is researching and writing about health topics, and I'm just as cynical as you about information based on rumor and hype. That's why, in my newsletter, just as in this book, I'll bring you honest, fully supported research to help you separate fact from fiction. In upcoming issues, I'll provide convincing information about:

* innovative ways to boost your energy—naturally
* enhancing your sex drive and saying no to Viagra
* updates on pain relief for arthritis sufferers
* exciting new weight loss supplements
* invigorating an aging or failing memory

Because I know you care about your health, I'm offering you the chance to receive a NO-RISK trial subscription to my monthly newsletter, *Health Watch*. Order today and start living a better, healthier life. If at any time you are not completely satisfied with my newsletter, you may simply cancel your subscription and receive a full refund.

As a preferred reader and someone who has already purchased one of my books, I'm offering this NO-RISK one-year trial subscription for only $36.95— or 38 percent off the regular subscription price of $59.95.

Healthfully yours,

Brenda D. Adderly

To order your NO-RISK trial subscription to my monthly *Health Watch* newsletter, call 1-888-211-2800, or send in the form below!

❏ YES! Please sign me up for my NO-RISK trial subscription to *Health Watch* for only $36.95 for 12 issues. I understand that I may cancel my subscription at any time and receive a full refund. Mail this card to: Alter-Net Health Technologies, 619 South June Street, Los Angeles, CA 90005. Allow four weeks for delivery.

❏ Visa   ❏ MC   ❏ AmEx   Expiration date: _____

Account no. _____

Please print: Mr./Mrs./Ms. _____

Address _____

City _____ State_____ Zip_____

Your signature _____